This Is Your Book That Will Help You Enhance Your Life

All-Natural and Complementary Therapies To Improve Your Well-Being

Rosa M. Altobelli

PAGE PUBLISHING
Conneaut Lake, PA

First originally published by Page Publishing 2022

ISBN 978-1-6624-8236-6 (pbk)
ISBN 978-1-6624-8237-3 (digital)

Printed in the United States of America

To my two angels at heaven, my husband, Orlando, and my son, Eddie, and you, friends, seeking for better quality of life.

Love, Rosa

Contents

Enjoy!

Introduction

This book does not dispense medical advice or prescribe the use of any technique as a replacement form of treatment for physical, mental, or medical problems by your doctor, either directly or indirectly.

My book's intention is to offer a variety of information and tools to help the readers in the quest for spiritual growth, emotional and physical well-being.

I wish with great humility to share all these natural therapies that help the mind, physical and spiritual, which, of course, does not replace the advice made by a medical doctor of your choice.

I want to tell you that I am not a naturist in the profession; everything you are going to read on these pages is from my own experience in life.

With my husband at twenty-three years old, we traveled to Yonkers, New York, from Buenos Aires, Argentina, newly married, to create a new life as well as seek more job opportunities.

Then we had the blessing of the birth of our son Eddie. We lived in Yonkers, New York, for eight years, then we moved to Torrance, California, where my husband did more the type of work that he was doing.

I started to have lots of muscle pains; the years passed, and I was still in a lot of body aches and felt depressed; the doctors prescribed a lot of medicine for me to take.

So I started to look for help through books and classes that could improve my health. Also, I read about the benefits of vitamins and minerals and doing a very nutritious diet, nourishing my body, and many of the natural and complementary therapies I will share in this book.

I was starting to feel a lot better, and that gave me the push to keep studying through wonderful books I picked up from the library and all the classes that I attended, like nutrition, yoga and meditation, learning to breathe properly, crystal healing, and aromatherapy with wonderful essential oils.

Acupressure and Reiki, a health care therapy, changed my life forever. I did all the levels of Reiki to become a teacher, and now I teach it to people who want to improve their life, relax, and enjoy life.

And that's why it is my honor to be able to transmit, through this humble book, these wonderful and complementary therapies to you, my dear friend. They help strengthen the mind, body, and emotional system.

I am going to introduce you first to aromatherapy; it's a therapeutic discipline that takes advantage of the property of essential oils to collaborate with the health and beauty of the human being.

For essential oils to acquire a therapeutic effect, they must be pure; this is very important. When buying them, make sure that the bottle says, "Organic and Therapeutic."

Unfortunately, low or adulterated oils that are on the market abound are not organic or therapeutic. It is better not to buy them since they can bring many problems to the skin and body.

I want to tell you that the first moment you open a bottle of essential oil, it's the moment you embark on an adventure that captivates you with all the senses that will occupy you all your life.

They lift your spirits or calm you down, removing all the stress of your day. There are many application methods: massages, compresses to relieve pains, also inhalation, air fresheners with a diffuser, and moisturizing creams for your face and body.

Several essential oils have contraindications for pregnant women and people with various allergies or with a health problem, such as hypertension or epilepsy.

In the case of children and the elderly, it is used in less proportion, and not all are recommended.

The Essential Oils

The essential oils that are not good for pregnant women or if you are breastfeeding the baby are *thyme, sage, cinnamon, cloves, juniper, rosemary, nutmeg, oregano, aniseeds,* and *fennel seeds.*

Please, please, inform yourself before purchasing. They are more essential oils that cannot be used in such cases.

Also, these oils should be avoided during the first three months of pregnancy: *chamomile, geranium, lavender,* and *rose.*

You also have to be very careful with these oils if you are going to go out in the sun or in a solar bed because they may stain your skin: *bergamot, orange, lemon, tangerine,* and all the citrus fruit.

Safe oils that do not need to be diluted are lavender and tea tree oil.

The base oil used for dilution of essential oils is sweet almond oil.

Coconut oil and jojoba oil is great as it not greasy; also grapeseed oil, argan oil, and olive oil.

It is very important that before you use the mixer, do a test on the inside of your arm with a little mix to be sure it's fine with you.

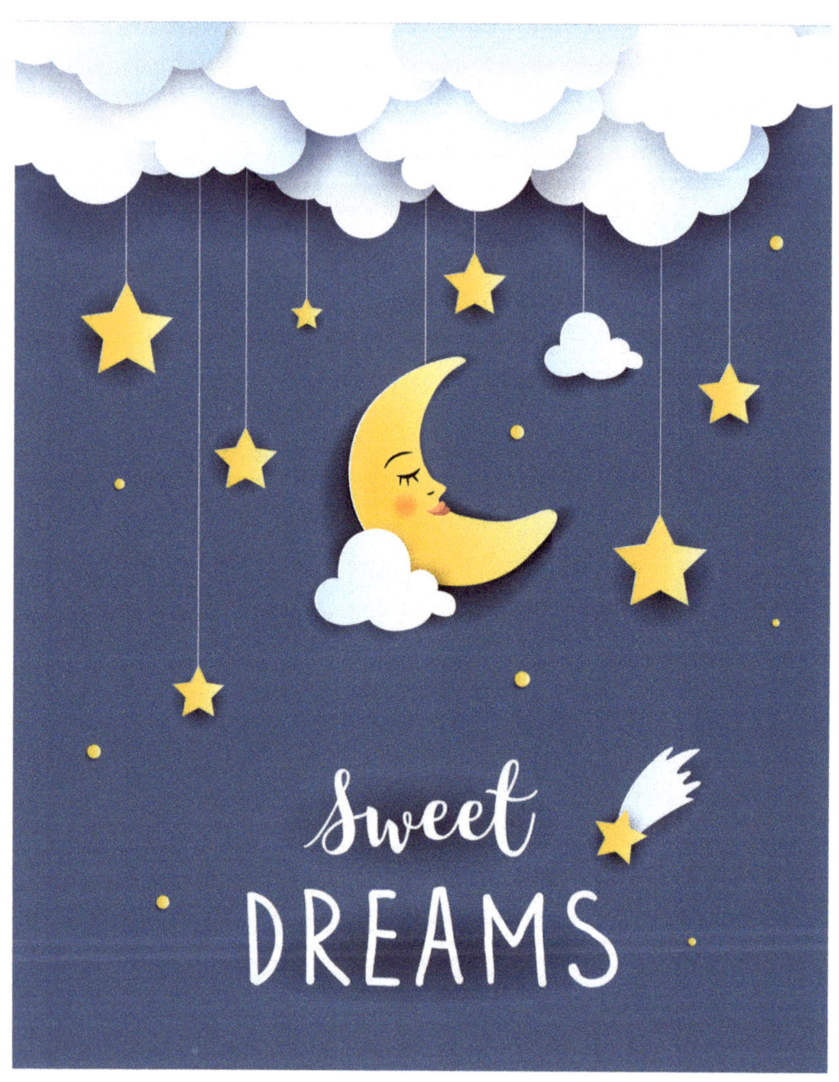
sweet
DREAMS

Recipe That Will Help You Have Pleasant Dreams

10 drops chamomile (essential oil)
5 drops sage (essential oil)
5 drops bergamot (essential oil)

Mix well and add 1 or 2 drops to a tissue that you put inside of the pillowcase.

*****

If you prefer to use an electric diffuser that carries water, you may like to put it on before going to bed.

2 drops chamomile (essential oil)
1 drop sage (essential oil)
1 drop bergamot (essential oil)

Note: If you put more than those drops, it can make a contradictory effect to the one you're looking for.

Dream Pillow

Here I am, offering you another idea that works very well to relax and loosen the muscles.

It's making a small pillow with a cotton cloth.

Cut 2 pieces of fabric, 8 inches and 6 inches. Sew all around, leaving a small opening to be able to fill it with these herbs or flowers.

Prepare 4 tablespoons lavender flowers, 2 tablespoon Melissa flower, and 2 tablespoons chamomile flowers. Plus, 3 tablespoon flax seeds and rose petals if you have them.

Sew the rest of the opening, and now you have warm company. You could heat it in a microwave for only 1 minute, or you can keep it in the freezer wrapped in a plastic bag so it doesn't smell like the frozen foods.

You can use this when you have a headache. This will relieve the pain a lot.

Note: Flax seeds are there to keep the dream pillow warm longer.

Enjoy.

Recipe for Muscle Aches in Morning

Mix 60 milliliters (4 tabs) of the base oil or neutral cream in a jar with 10 drops rosemary (essential oil), 8 drops eucalyptus (essential oil), 6 drops cypress (essential oil), 3 drops thyme essential oil), and 3 drops peppermint (essential oil).

Mix everything and apply to where the pains are.

*****

For Muscle Pains to Apply at Night

Mix in a jar 60 milliliters (4 tabs) base oil or neutral cream with 10 drops chamomile (essential oil), 10 drops sage (essential oil), 4 drops coriander (essential oil), 4 drops cypress (essential oil), and 4 drops ylang-ylang (essential oil).

Mix everything and apply to where the pains are.

Sweet Dreams

Useful Conversion Guide

1 mL. = 20 drops of essential oil
5 mL. =1 tsp. carrier oil
25 mL. =5 tsp.
30 mL. =2 tbs. = 1 fl. oz. = 600 drops
40 mL. =8 tsp. carrier oil or base lotion for massage
20 mL. =4 tsps. of base oil
35 mL. =6 1/2 tsp.
1 cc. = 20 drops
5 cc. = 1 tsp. = 100 drops
10 cc. = 2 tsps. = 200 drops
15 cc. = 1 tbs. = 300 drops
100 mL. almond oil = 20 tsp.
1/2 eyedropper holds approximately 10 drops
1 eyedropper holds 20 drops
1 oz. bottle = 30 cc. = 2 tbs.
2 oz. bottle = 60 cc. = 4 tabs = 1,200 drops
4 oz. bottle =120 cc. = 1/2 c. = 8 tbs or 2,400 drops
8 oz. = 240 c. = 1 c. = 16 tbs. = 3,600 drops

Note: The ratio of essential oils to carrier oil is 5 drops essential oils in 10 milliliters (10 ounces) or 2 teaspoons carrier oils enough for body massage; it is 2.5 percent dilution.

For example, if you have 30 milliliters, 10 ounces bottle of carrier oil, you will need to add 15 drops of essential oil, or for 50 milliliters or 2 ounces jar, add 25 drops of essential oil.

Aromatherapy and Your Body

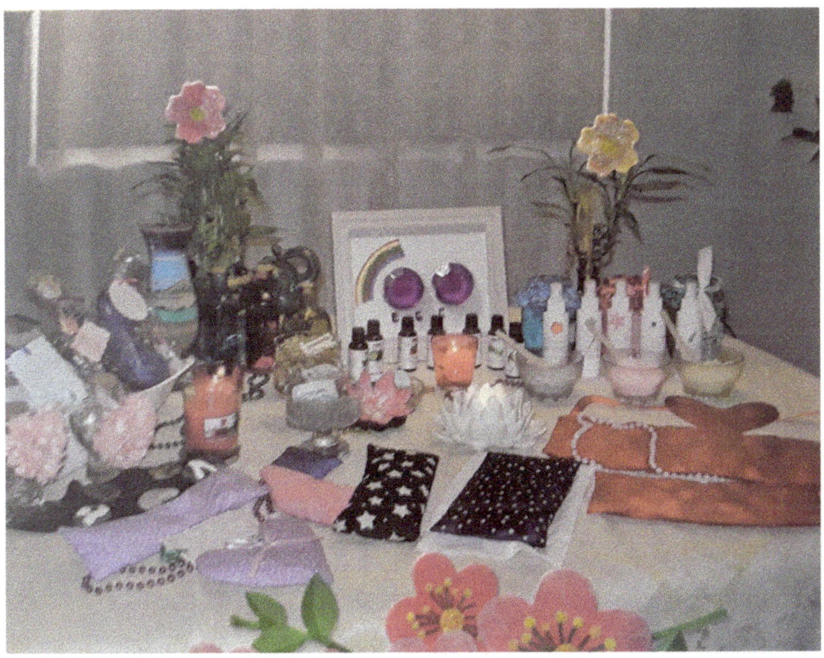

The ingredients of essential oils can ease muscle tension, improve your mood, boost your circulation, and clear respiratory problems, such as stuffy nose and sore throats. By rubbing your oils over or onto the affected area.

To release a blocked nose, very good oils are peppermint, rosemary, eucalyptus, and lavender; all are very beneficial oils.

To ease sore throat, frankincense, sandalwood, and jasmine oil.

To ease eczema, chamomile, juniper berry, lavender, and also, geranium.

To improve cellulite, juniper berry, geranium, and also, rosemary

To relax sore and aching muscles, ginger, sweet marjoram, rosemary, and also, very good frankincense.

To relax stomach and period pains, clary sage, aniseed, lavender, and marjoram.

To ease upset stomachs, ginger, peppermint, and tangerine.
To moisturize dry skin, rose, sandalwood, ylang-ylang, and chamomile.
To help oily skin, cypress, lemon, and tea tree oil (also good for acne).

Note: Undiluted essential oils can be used in vaporizers.

Dilute up to 10 drops essential oil to 30 milliliters (2 tablespoons) carrier oil of your preference before using it on your skin.

Enjoy!

Vaporizing Essential Oils

Vaporizers may be used anywhere in the home or office. They can help lift your spirit and relax you after a hard day's work. Their effects are subtle and are better suited to raising your mood a little than healing or focusing your concentration during meditation.

- Create a relaxing mood using a candle vaporizer.
- Surround it with scented candles for a more intense experience.
- Candle vaporizers consist of a small bowl of oil and water suspended over a candle. The heat from the candle causes the oil to evaporate into the air. Fill the vaporizer bowl with water and add three to five drops of the essential oil that you like.
- As a candle vaporizer doesn't need electricity, it can be used anywhere; you can use undiluted essential oils in a vaporizer or buy a special vaporizer blend. In both cases, you need to add up to five drops to the vaporizer bowl.

Please note that oils that are already blended for use in massage are usually not suitable for use in vaporizers. The best essential oils to use in your vaporizer are

- for relaxing, lavender, mandarin, sweet marjoram, and melissa;
- for energizing, lemon, bergamot, rosemary, and peppermint;
- for headaches, chamomile, lavender, neroli, marjoram, and rosemary;
- for antiseptic, eucalyptus, tree tea, thyme, and juniper berry; and
- for sensual, lavender, ylang-ylang, and rose.

Personal Mixture to Tune the Nerves

2 tbs. jojoba oil
4 drops lavender (essential oil)
3 drops clary sage (essential oil)
3 drops sandalwood (essential oil)
2 drops neroli (essential oil)
1 drop vetiver (essential oil)

Add the essential oils to the jojoba oil and mix well; use this formula as a fragrance or inhale directly from the bottle as needed.

*****

Personal Floral Mixture to Preventive Panic Attacks

2 tbs. jojoba oil
4 drops geranium (essential oil)
2 drops chamomile (essential oil)
2 drops lavender (essential oil)
1 drop jasmine absolute (essential oil)
1 drop neroli (essential oil)
1 drop ylang-ylang (essential oil)

Mix all the ingredients and use as a fragrance or inhale as needed.

You always have to do a little test to be sure you don't have an allergy to the mix of essential oils that you made. Don't overlook these important steps; it's your body and skin.

I want to tell you something very nice and important about the essential oils.

When we inhale the oils, the smell molecules transmit to the emotional centers of the brain called the limbic system. This system is connected to other parts of the brain that are wrapped with memory, breathing, blood circulation, and also, the endocrine glands, which regulate the level of hormones in the body.

I tell you; the moment you open a bottle of the essential oil, you will embark on an adventure that captivates all your senses that will occupy you all your life. They lift your spirit or soothe you by removing the stress the whole day.

Enjoy them!

This Recipe Is for People Who Suffer from Restless Legs

During the night, this recipe will help you relax them and be able to sleep better.

In a small bottle with a fine spray top, place 1 cup of distilled water with 12 drops of lavender (essential oil). Use before going to bed; shake well before spraying it on your legs.

*****

A Mix to Spray Pillows and Sheets
Recipe to Help You Have Pleasant Sleep

A small bottle with a fine spray top
1/2 cup distilled water with 7 drops lavender (essential oil)
2 drops melissa (essential oil)
1 drop sage (essential oil)
Mix and shake well before use.

Sweet dreams!

Recipes That Help Lower Anxiety and Panic Attacks

Mix 3 tbs. vegetable oil with 10 drops lavender (essential oil)
6 drops ylang-ylang (essential oil)
4 drops frankincense (essential oil)
2 drops chamomile (essential oil)
1 drop sage (essential oil)

Mix with a wooden spoon and place in a glass bottle. Use on your wrist, neck, and temples.

Note: This mixture relaxes you a lot; don't go out driving while using this mix.

*****

Recipe for Headache Pain and Relaxation

Mix 1 tbs. vegetable or sweet almond oil
10 drops lavender (essential oil)
5 drops peppermint (essential oil)
2 drops chamomile (essential oil)
1 capsule vitamin E (200 mg)

Mix gently and use it when you have a headache and pain in your temples. For head and back of the head.

Enjoy!

Another Recipe to Take with You on Your Purse or for the Office That Is for Headaches

Mix 30 milliliters (2 tablespoons) of neutral gel inside a roll-on bottle with 5 drops of mint (essential oil) with 3 drops of lemongrass. Mix gently and enjoy this mixture before the first symptoms.

Use in your temples and on the back of your head.

*****

Recipe for Depression or low Concentration

Use it on the bottom of your feet.

Mix 3 tbs. cream or carrier oil
6 drops sandalwood (essential oil)
4 drops ylang-ylang (essential oil)
3 drops tangerine or mandarin (essential oil)
3 drops geranium (essential oil)
1 drop neroli (essential oil)

Mix for Serenity

Mix in 1 cup of distilled water in a bottle with a vaporizer top.

20 drops mandarin (essential oil)
10 drops lavender (essential oil)
5 drops sandalwood (essential oil)

Shake before use and spray the room when you want everyone to be relax, including the children.

*****

Recipe for a Focused Mind

For studying, taking an exam, or to be more alert.

Mix 1/2 cup distilled water in a small bottle so that you can spray the place. This will help you study in better concentration and when you want to be more alert.

Mix the water with 10 drops peppermint (essential oil) with 10 drops rosemary (essential oil). Mix gently and enjoy.

Tonic for the Skin of Roses
(Or for Room Spray)

Glass container
250 mL. water
10 drops cereal alcohol
Rose petals from one rose
Paper filter

Place in the container the water, add one by one the petals of the rose and add cereal alcohol. The cereal alcohol serves as a preservative; let stand well covered for a week. Place through a paper filter. Spray your skin, or you can perfume the home with the aroma of roses that it generates. Harmony, Tranquility, and a lot of well-being.

*****

Sanitizing Gel for Compulsive Disorders
Combat Anxiety and Regain Harmony

3 tbs. gel alcohol
4 drops patchouli (essential oil)
4 drops petitgrain (essential oil)

Incorporate in a container with a vaporizer. Let stand for a few days.

The gel not only acts as an antiseptic but also as aromatherapy. This helps people who suffer from obsessive disorders that fear spreading and coming into contact with others.

Soothing Massage Oil

Pour 4 tablespoons of almond oil into a glass bottle with a stopper and add 10 drops lavender, 5 drops clary sage, and 5 drops chamomile (essential oils). Mix gently to mix all ingredients; store the bottle in a dark, cool place.

Note: Before use, do a patch test.
(Although generally safe to use clary sage and chamomile oils. It should be avoided during pregnancy.)

*****

Seductive Massage Oil

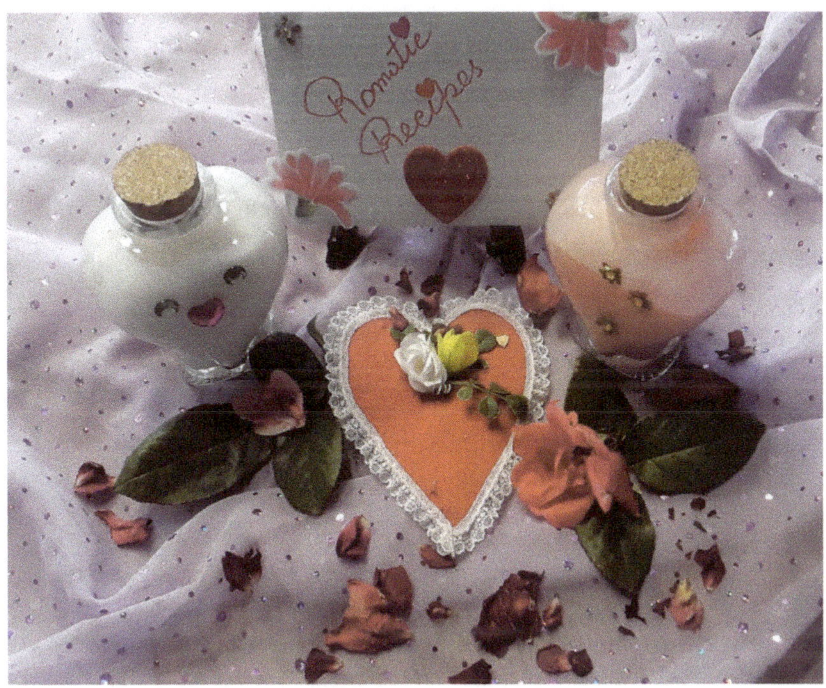

Enough for three full-body massages.

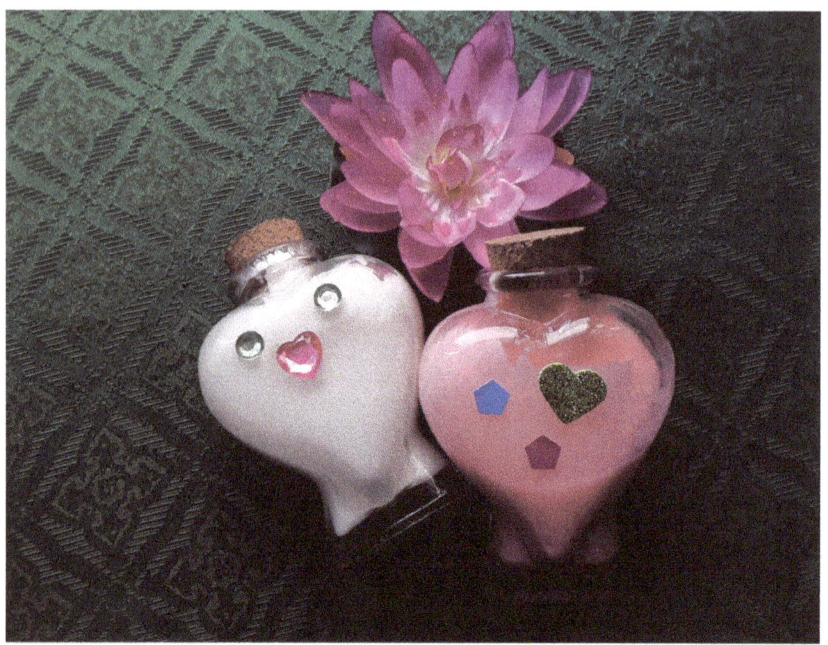

50 mL. (3 tbs.) almond oil
15 drops rose (essential oils)
5 drops coriander (essential oils)
2 drops cedarwood (essential oils)
Mix gently and enjoy body massage.

Baby Care Infant Massage Oil

1/4 ounce (1/2 tbs.) aloe vera oil
1/2 ounce (1 tbs.) almond oil

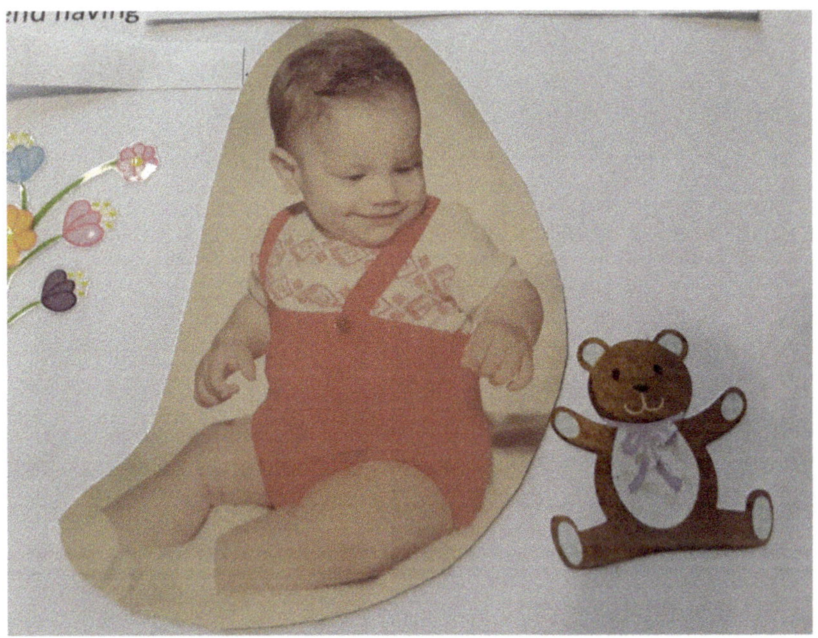

1/4 oz (1/2 tbs.) hazelnut oil

Essential Oils:
3 drops blue chamomile
7 drops lavender
Makes one ounce (2 tbs.)

When the baby needs an extra boost for the immune system and calming down, I recommend having the aroma around them rather than using the oils on their skin directly.

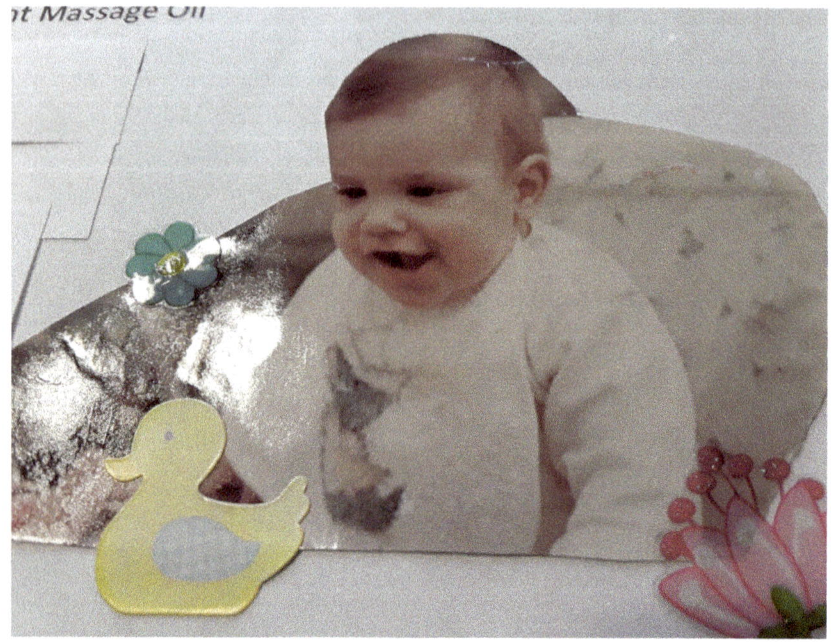

Energizing and Slenderizing Body Oil

4 oz (1/2 cup) of sunflower or canola oil
10 drops rosemary (essential oil)
10 drops lemon (essential oil)
10 drops orange (essential oil)
5 drops basil (essential oil)
3 drops peppermint (essential oil)

Blend and put in a decorative bottle.

*****

Basic Cellulitis Bath to Help Rid of Excess Body Fluids

1 cup sea salt
1/2 cup baking soda
1 1/2 cup Epsom salt
3 drops cypress (essential oil)
3 drops lemon (essential oil)
1 drop juniper (essential oil)

Pour in the warm water; mix well before you go into the bathtub.

Gentle Face Scrub (Enough for Ten Treatments)

3 tbs. almond oil in a glass bowl
3 tbs. oatmeal
3 tbs. powdered milk
2 tbs. powered rose petals

Mix all ingredients together and store in a sealed jar.

Before using, mix to a soft paste with the almond oil and gently rub it on your skin with light touches using circular motions. Be careful around the delicate areas of the eyes. Rinse off with warm water and pat your face dry.

*****

Gentle Face Mask for One Treatment

This mix of oatmeal, egg, and honey soothes and nourishes the skin while gently lifting impurities from your skin.

4 tbs. fine oatmeal
1 egg yolk
1 tbs. runny honey

Mix the honey and egg yolk together and slowly add the oatmeal to make a soft paste. Use immediately; smooth the mask on the skin and leave for 15 minutes. Rinse off with lukewarm water and pat dry.

Recipe to Balance and Rejuvenate the Complexion

This is a low dilution for sensitive skin.

Blend in 4 teaspoons (20 mL.) carrier oil as jojoba or almond oil with 3 drops palma rose and 2 drops roman chamomile (essential oil). Apply as needed.

*****

Add Up the Previous Recipe

4 drops palma rose (essential oil)
3 drops frankincense (essential oil)
3 drops sandalwood (essential oil)
Mix and massage gently to your face especially at night.

Enjoy!

Massage Oil to Stimulate Immunity

120 mL. (8 tbs.) base oil
10 drops geranium (essential oil)
10 drops tea tree (essential oil)
8 drops lemon (essential oil)
6 drops myrrh (essential oil)

Pour the base oil into a clean bowl and add the essential oils, and gently mix. Once to twice a day, massage your body with this mix.

Improve the Immune System

Morning Bath to Strengthen Immunity

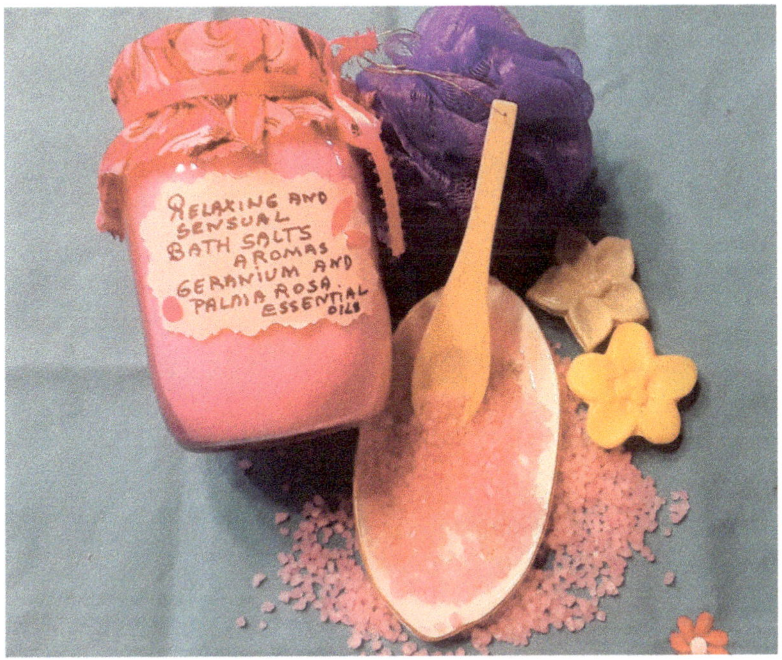

4 drops tea tree (essential oil)
3 drops rosemary (essential oil)
2 drops lemon (essential oil)
1 drop ginger (essential oil)

Disperse the oils in the bathtub and immerse yourself for 15 to 20 minutes.

Night Bath to Strengthen Immunity

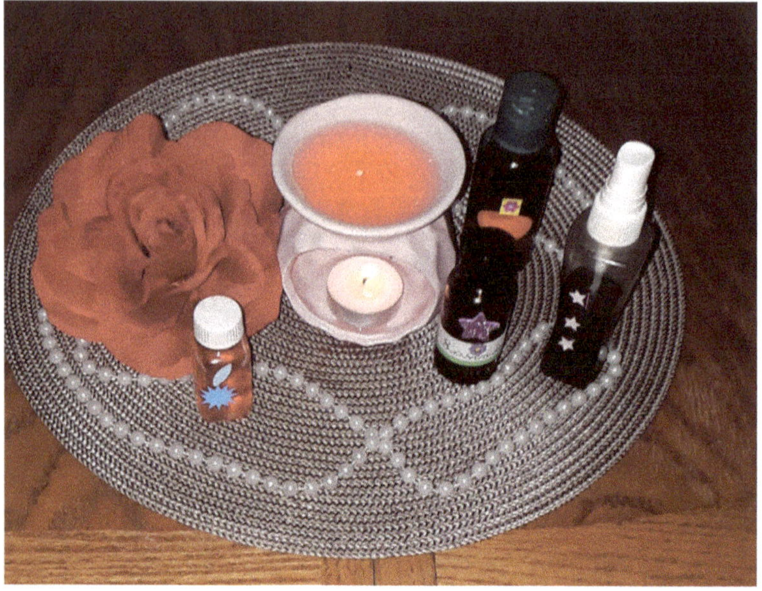

4 drops tea tree (essential oil)
2 drops sage (essential oil)
2 drops orange (essential oil)
2 drops rosewood (essential oil)

Disperse the oils in the bathtub with warm water in the early hours of the night or before bedtime and immerse in this wonderful mix for 15 to 20 minutes.

Citrus Sanitizing Spray for Home

20 drops lemon (essential oils)
20 drops orange (essential oils)
15 drops bergamot (essential oils)
5 drops lime (essential oils)
1 bottle (4 oz.) with spray cap.

Fill the bottle with 3 ounces water and 1 ounce perfume alcohol or vodka. Add the essential oils one at a time to the mix. Cap the bottle and shake well before using.

Note: You may use white distilled vinegar instead of alcohol.

Herbal Facial Hydrosol

1 c. distilled water
2 drops rosemary (essential oils)
2 drops clary sage (essential oils)
2 drops chamomile (essential oils)

Blend together in a decorative or colored glass spray bottle. Shake well before use. *Not for your eyes.*

*****

Floral Spray for All Kinds of Skin Type

8 tbs. distilled water into an atomizer bottle
3 drops lavender (essential oils)
2 drops rosewood (essential oils)
1 drop chamomile (essential oils)
1 drop rose (essential oils)

Shake gently and spray on your skin several times a day.

Note: Not for your eyes.

Aftershave Lotion for All Skin Types

240 mL. (16 tbs.) distilled water
2 drops cedar (essential oils)
2 drops lavender (essential oils)
2 drops rosewood (essential oils)
2 drops vetiver (essential oils)

Shake well; wet your face with this formula and shake before each application.

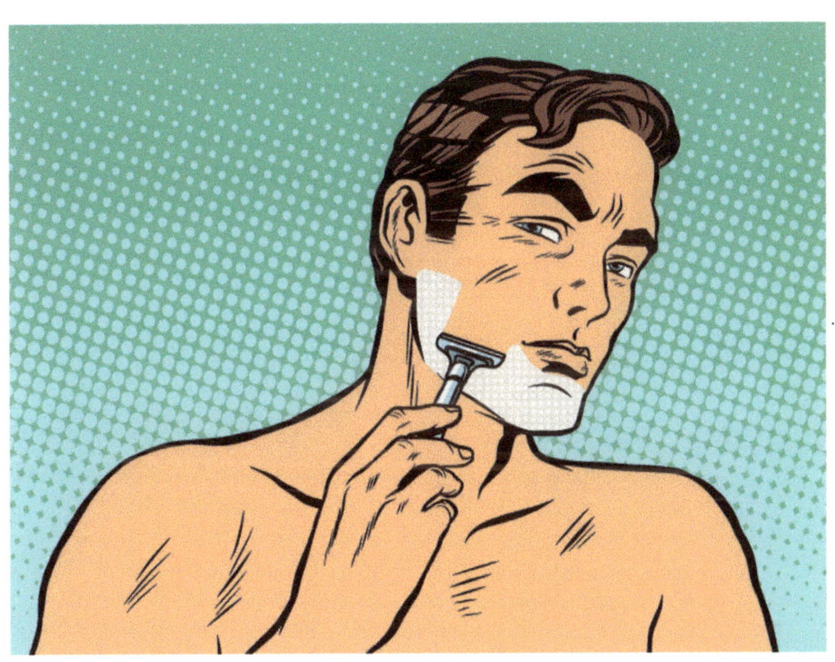

Emulsion for After Shaving

175 mL. (12 tbs.) coconut oil
6 tbs. almond oil
1/2 cucumber
4 drops sandalwood (essential oils)
4 drops lavender (essential oils)

Melt the coconut oil in a simmered container and remove it from the stove. Add the almond oil, peel the 1/2 cucumber, and liquefy, strain the obtained mix and mix well. Place in a jar with a screw cap or watertight closure.

Eau de Cologne for Men

2 to 4 oz. bottle with lid
6 drops grapefruit (essential oils)
5 drops sweet orange (essential oils)
2 drops cypress (essential oils)
2 drops sandalwood (essential oils)
2 drops lavender (essential oils)

Fill the bottle with perfume, alcohol, or vodka. Mix well and rest for a week before used. All the essential oils have protective properties.

Enjoy!

*****

Recipe for Knee Pain

4 oz. carrier oil
24 drops peppermint (essential oils)
24 drops eucalyptus (essential oils)

Both oils have an anesthetic and anti-inflammatory properties that are ideal on treating sore joints. Massage with a small portion of this mix on painful areas.

What Are Chakras?

Chakras are the energy center of the body; a Sanskrit word *chakra* means wheel or disk, and each chakra moves with a spinning motion, forming a vortex.

It is this vortex that filters the energy of the environment around us and disperses it throughout our bodies. They are seven major chakras that enter the physical body, at the top of the head and the other six.

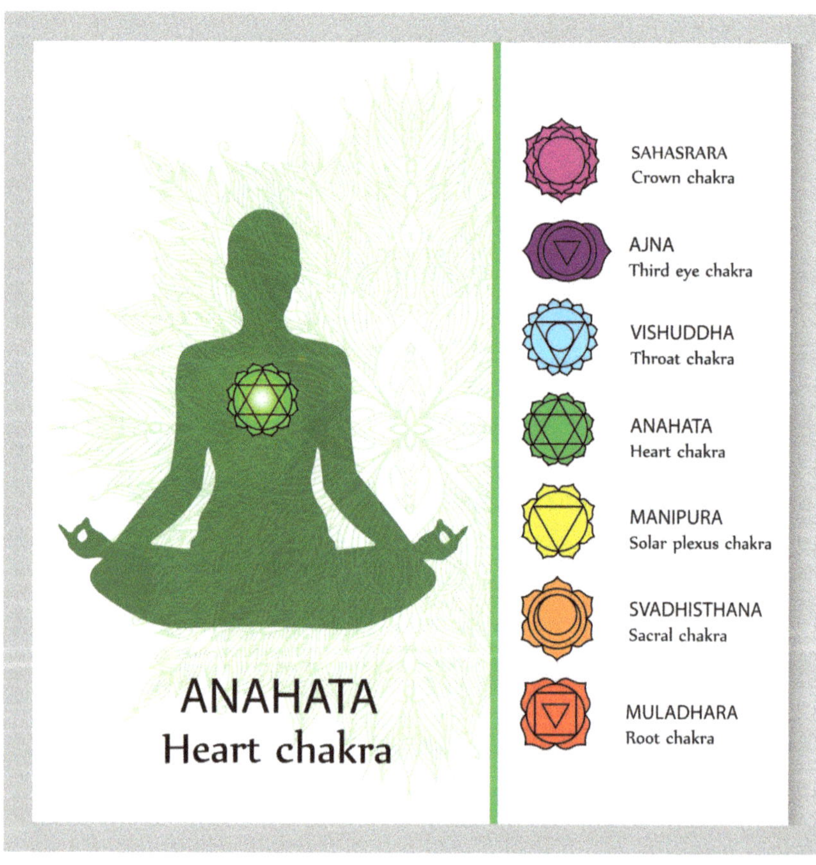

Along the vertical midline of the body, it is important to remember that the chakras are constantly interacting and that they are no more separate from each other than they are from our aura. Our body's seven energy centers are the gateways to that spiritual growth of the person; if we understand how these centers work, we can work with them to bring our body, mind, and emotions back into balance with our true nature.

As each energy center spins, it emanates its own unique frequency and color that keys into one of the seven rainbow rays of light; when an energy center is blocked, we can experience fatigue, health problems, emotional imbalance, and lethargy.

When energy is flowing freely through an energy center, we feel energetic, creative, and at peace. The energy created from our emotions and mental attitude runs through the chakras and is distributed to our cells and tissue organs. Realizing this brings tremendous insight into how we, ourselves, affect our bodies, mind, and circumstances for better or worst.

Experience and understand that chakras mean that you understand the fly of life, including the meaning of life and death. You might possess the most precious gems, yet if you don't know their value, then there is no difference between the gem and an ordinary pebble.

Chakras

Crown Chakra

Highest chakra symbolizing the merging of the human mind with the divine.

Location: top and center of the head
Body Associations: brain, cerebellum, and pineal gland
Colors: violet and white

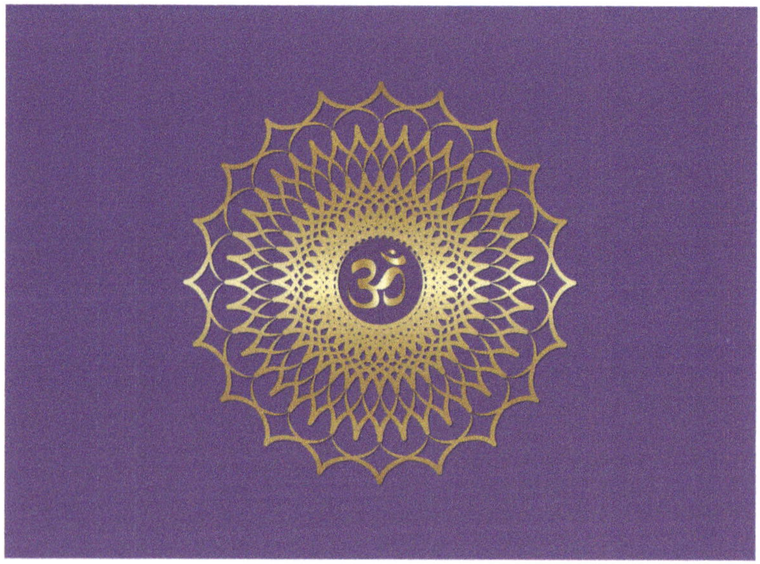

Scents: frankincense and lotus
Gemstones: amethyst, clear quartz, and sugilite.
Zodiac: Capricorn and Pisces

Third Eye Chakra

Center of creativity, intuition, insight, and devotion to spiritual knowledge.

Location: between the eyes

AJNA
third eye chakra

Body Associations: face, eyes, nose, sinus, pituitary and pineal glands
Colors: indigo
Scents: jasmine, vetiver, mint gemstones, and lapis sodalite
Zodiac: Sagittarius, Aquarius, and Pisces

Throat Chakra

Center of communication, speech, effect of the spoken word on truth, knowledge, wisdom, and kindness.

Location: between collarbones
Body Associations: upper lungs, bronchioles, esophagus, trachea, vocal cords, throat, thyroid, neck, ears, and arms
Colors: light sky blue
Scents: neroli, sage, and eucalyptus
Gemstones: aquamarine, turquoise, and chalcedony
Zodiac: Gemini, Aquarius, and Taurus

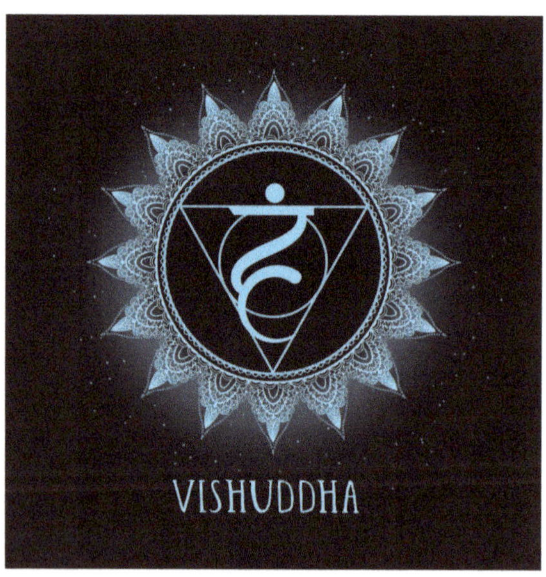

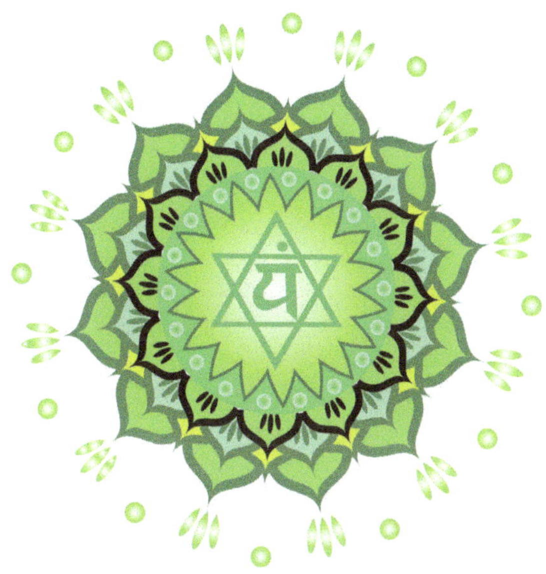

Heart Chakra

Center of compassion, altruism, forgiveness, and acceptance of reality as it is.

Location: center of the chest
Body Associations: heart, upper back, lower lungs, breasts, and blood
Color: green
Scents: rose, geranium gemstones, rose quartz, green jade, pink tourmaline, kunzite, and emerald
Zodiac: Leo and Libra

Solar Plexus Chakra

Center of self-respect, willpower, confidence, and physical energy

Location: alightly down from the navel
Body Associations: lower back, abdomen, digestive organs, liver, gall-bladder, spleen, and autonomic nervous system
Colors: sunny yellow
Scents: lavender, rosemary, and bergamot
Gemstones: tiger eye, amber citrine, topaz, and gold

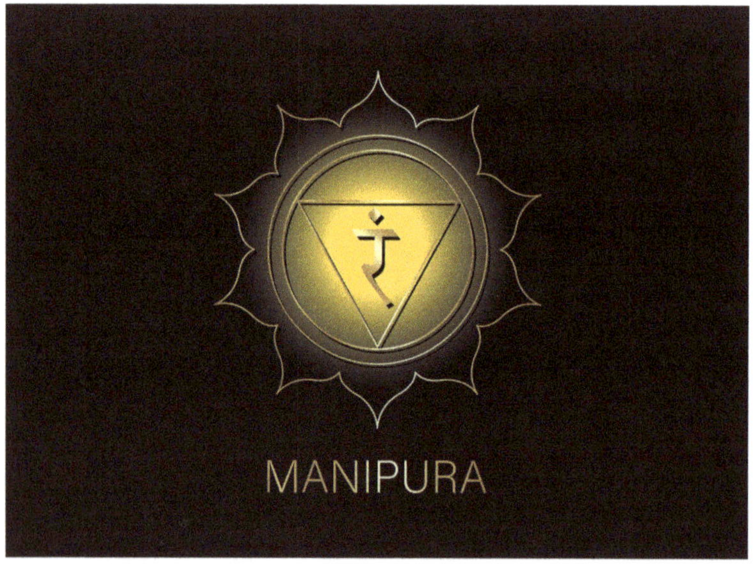

Zodiac: Leo, Sagitarias, and Virgo

Sacral Chakra

Center of feeling, emotion, sexual desire, craving, family life, harmony, and tolerance

Location: slightly above genital area

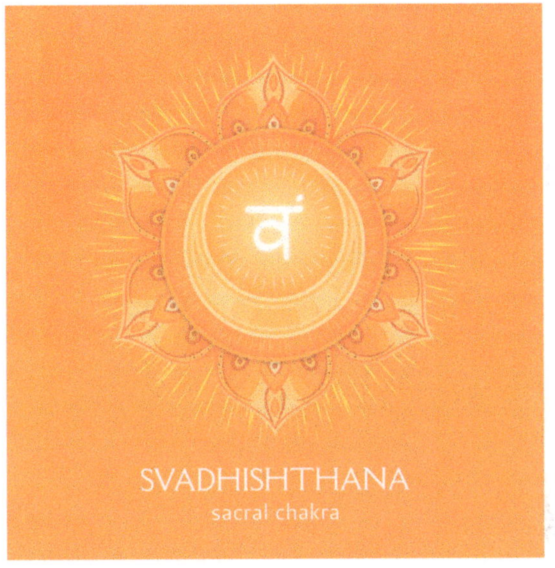

Body Associations: reproductive organs, kidneys, bladder, pelvic girdle, blood, and lymph

Colors: orange
Scents: ylang-ylang and sandalwood
Gemstones: carnelian and moonstone
Zodiac: Cancer, Libra, and Scorpio

Root Chakra

Center of the basic will to survive and material world. Courage, stability, and physical health.

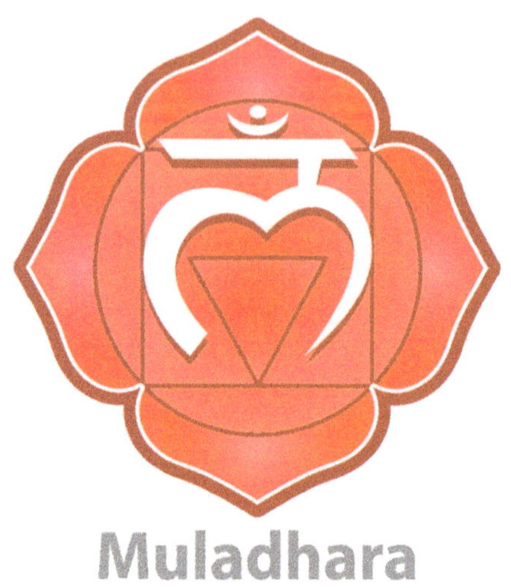

Location: between genitals and anus.
Body Associations: all solid parts, spinal column, bones, teeth, anus, rectum, colon, prostate, blood, and cells
Colors: vibrant red
Scents: cedar and clove.
Gemstones: agate, hematite, and blood jasper.
Zodiac: Aries, Taurus, Scorpio, and Capricorn

CHAKRAS

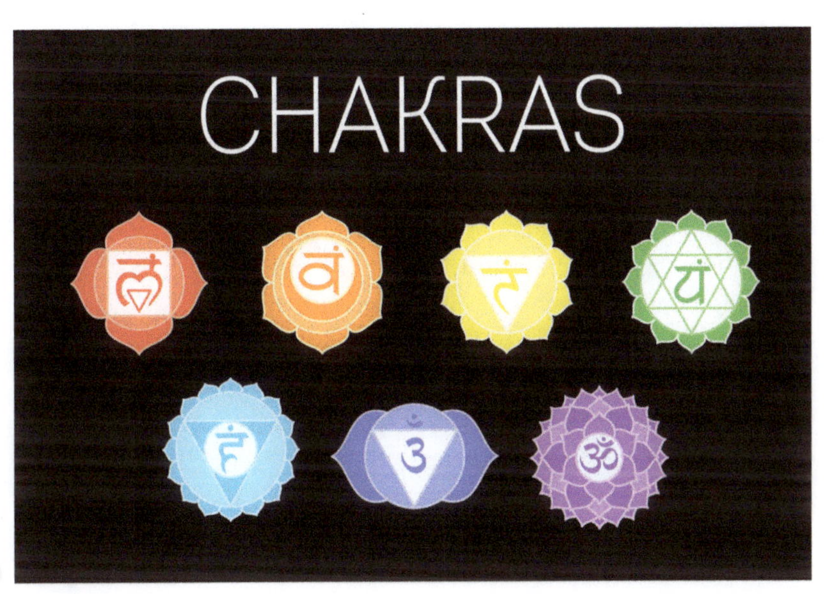

The Feet Chakras

The feet chakras are the chakras of the base, the ones that keep us with the feet on the ground. We feel out of reality because, normally, the chakras of the feet are de-energized (cold).

The colors of the feet chakras are black and smoky since black is good to help the person return to acquire security in himself and knows what he wants.

Good to use a hematite stone or smoky quartz on each foot when you are doing a healing session, such as Reiki or crystal healing.

The Hands Chakras

The hand chakras are located in the center of the palms of the hands. They are linked with the white or transparent color because they make the conductors of the energy of light or energy of healing.

Through the chakras of the hands, we will channel the energy of our intuition, placing some crystals that we have chosen in our body or in another person. We will use a Crystal Quartz and the colors of the seven chakras in the body during a healing session.

Namaste!

Dietary Guidelines for Nourishing Your Energy Centers

When you think about your chakra's system, you probably aren't considering the type of food that you eat that can help you nourish your chakras. It is important to feed and nourish the flesh in order to help support and fuel our chakras.

Whenever one or more of your chakras is misaligned, you might do well to look and see if you are not eating or possibly overeating the foods that fuel that particular chakra.

Feeding Your Root Chakra (Grounding)

- Root vegetables such as carrots, potatoes, radishes, garlic, onions, etc.
- Protein rich foods: eggs, meats, beans, tofu, and peanut butter.
- Spices: horseradish, hot paprika, chives, cayenne and pepper.

Feeding Your Sacral Chakra

- Nourishing the sexual creativity center, sweet fruits, passion fruit, coconut and honey.
- Nuts such as almonds, walnuts, etc.
- Spices: cinnamon, vanilla, carob, sweet paprika, and sesame seeds.

Feeding Your Solar Plexus Chakra

- Boosting self-esteem and encouraging self-love.
- Granola and grains, pastas, breads, cereals, rice, flax seeds, and sunflower seeds.
- Dairy: milk, cheese, and yogurt.
- Spices: ginger, mints, spearmint, melissa, chamomile, turmeric, and fennel.

Feeding Your Heart Chakra

- Healing emotional pains.
- Leafy vegetables: broccoli, cauliflower, cabbage, celery, squash, etc.
- Liquids: green teas.
- Spices: basil, sage, thyme, cilantro, and parsley.

Feeding Your Throat Chakra

- Speaking one's truth.
- Liquids in general: water, fruit juices, and herbal teas.
- Tart or tangy fruits: lemons, limes, grapefruit, and kiwi.
- Other tree growing fruits: apples, pears, plums, peaches, apricots, etc.
- Spices: salt and lemon grass.

Feeding Your Brow Chakra

- Awakening third eye senses.
- Dark bluish-colored fruits: blueberries, red grapes, black-berries, raspberries, etc.
- Liquids: red wine and grape juice.
- Spices: lavender, poppy seed, and mugwort.

Feeding Your Crown Chakra

- Opening and clearing the spiritual communication center.
- Air: fasting and detoxing your body.
- Incense and smudging herbs: sage, copal, myrrh, frankin-cense, and juniper (incense and smudging herbs not to be eaten but are ritually inhaled through the nostrils).

The Crystals

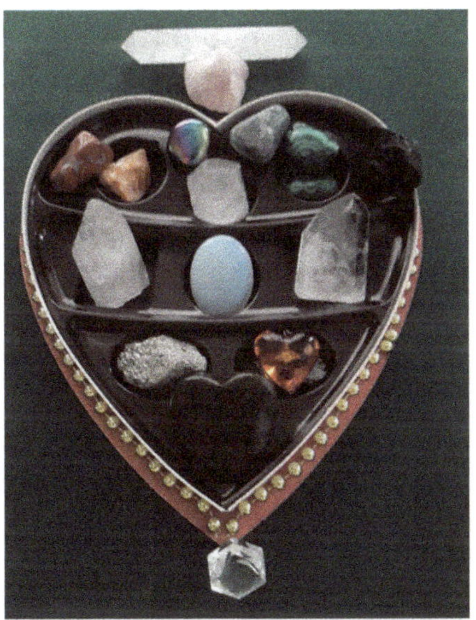

This chapter is dedicated to the wonderful wonders of nature.

You will find on these pages crystals that will help you calm your anxiety, help with emotions, help you meditate to give you self-confidence, and much more.

I will mention some of them, but I am sure you will be very interested in looking deeper into the natural wonders that our wonderful earth has provided to help us be happier in our life. Enjoy them and treasure their wisdom.

The most common crystal to find is the amethyst, the anxiety crystal for stress. It calms the mind with the beautiful purple color. Amethyst and rose quartz are very good friends to help you sleep.

While the purple of the Amethyst calms the mind, the soft rose quartz soothes the heart, which is vital for a peaceful sleep. These two wonderful crystals will assist you in maintaining the energy you need to sleep better.

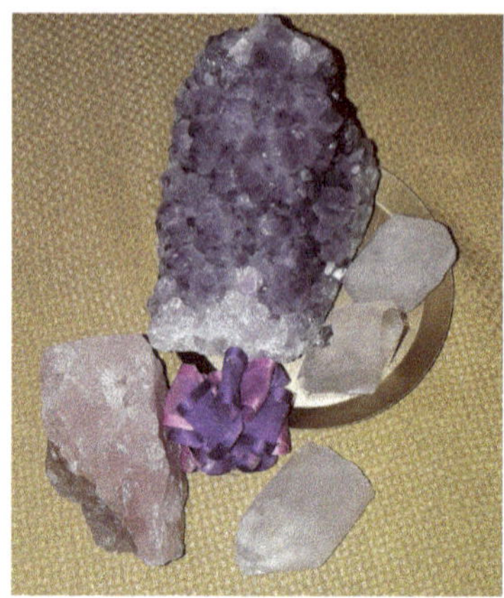

Selecting the crystals you want and taking care of them is an important part of building a collection.

This can become a very rewarding pastime as well as have interesting subtle effects on your living space and your life. Crystals have their own *frequency* thanks to the arrangement of their molecules, and so do you.

If you feel the attraction to get a stone or a crystal, it is because the crystal picked you first. When you buy a crystal, it is a good idea to clean them before using it. Cleansing is not just about removing dirt, grease, and dust; it is also to clear previous energies from the stone.

Simply hold your crystal under flowing cold water for several minutes and visualize all other energy traces being dissolved. Crystals should be cleaned regularly, especially if they are used for healing.

The Crystals That Will Add a Sparkle to Your Life

Rose quartz, green aventurine, ruby gemstone, rhodochrosite, carnelian, agate garnet, etc.

These crystals and stones could be used as a carrier or worn as jewelry, as a pendant necklace, a bracelet, or under your pillow to maintain mental clarity.

Purple and indigo crystals such as amethyst, labradorite, and sodalite share the soothing properties of lavender; combine them with the dried herb in a healing talisman to ease headaches.

Clear crystals, such as white quartz, share the cleansing properties of the white flowers, such as roses; combine them to keep the atmosphere pure.

You can use a crystal healing wand or smaller polisher stones to channel healing energy into your body. Rub or *anoint* your crystals with complementary essential oils to boost their healing and protective abilities.

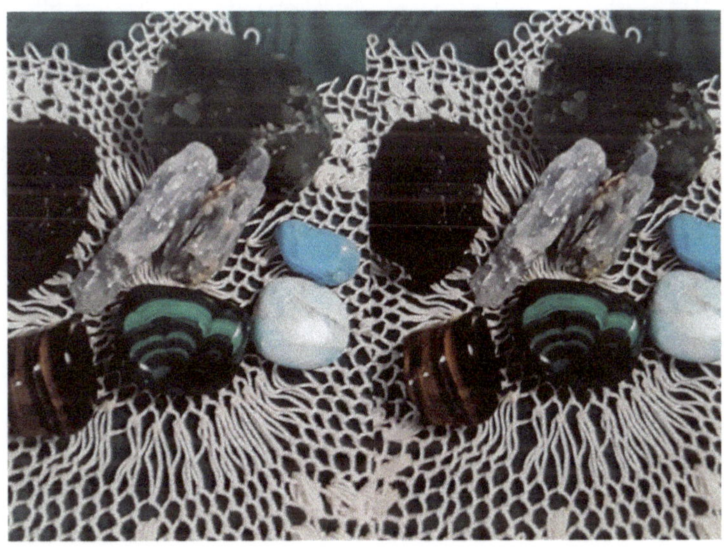

Carnelian is an orange-red or pink feel-better stone. It helps with study, memory, and inspiration; it can relieve apathy and bring vitality and self-esteem, etc. It is very good for digestion and revitalizing the blood, and much more.

Citrine is a yellow golden variety that they call the "money stone." It brings abundance and wealth; it is very good for anemia, decision, creativity, awareness, writing, and a new beginning.

Green jade is very good for healing emotional issues and brings peace to both inner and outer health and helps a lot with the physical body, such as skin, lymphatic system, wisdom, compassion, etc.

Rose quartz and rhodochrosite are beautiful stones from Argentina. It calms the heart chakra with love, like a bubble bath for emotions.

Sodalite is good for calming mental health, healing, and communicating with feelings.

Lapis lazuli is a feel-better stone that brings vitality, wisdom, and creative expression.

Malachite is good for physical balance, encourages restful sleep, and helps with pains.

Crystals Care

Many crystals are friable; crystals that are layered or clustered can separate, such as selenite are water-soluble. Polished surfaces or natural points are easily scratched or damaged.

Tumble stones are more durable. When not in use, wrap your crystals in a silk or velvet little bag. This prevents scratching and protects the crystals against absorbing foreign energies.

Crystals need to be cleaned when you buy them and after wearing or using them for healing. A few crystals never need cleansing, such as citrine, kyanite, clear quartz, and carnelian cleanse others crystals.

The tumble stones can be kept in a pretty small bag.

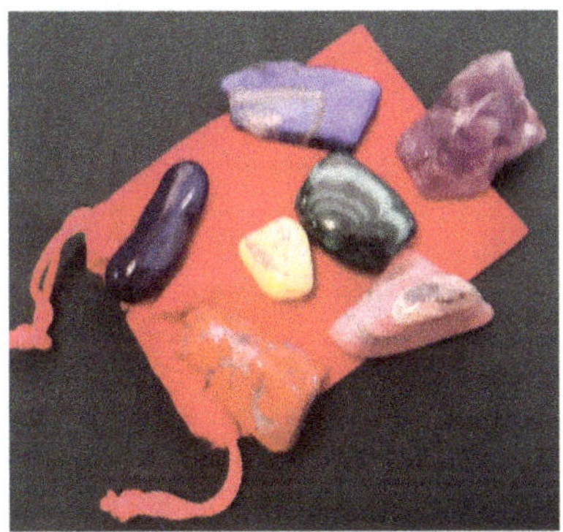

One of the easiest ways to clean, purify, and reenergize is to use water and sea salt; you can *smudge* them and visualize them (surround white light around your crystal) in the earth (in clean soil for twenty-four hours).

They are various crystals that are very special in meditations. Meditating with crystals is one of the easiest ways to tune to its energy. Start with the red crystal to energize and awaken.

Then with orange stone, such as Citrine, then with green one, there are so many crystals. Look for the one that attracts you. Also, blue, such as celestine, an angel stone, and purple and black stones like tourmaline, obsidian, etc.

They are very grounding, and don't forget the "universal healer," the white quartz. I personally meditate with *apophyllite* crystal that I love very much. Apophyllite crystals can enhance your psychic vision and clairvoyance.

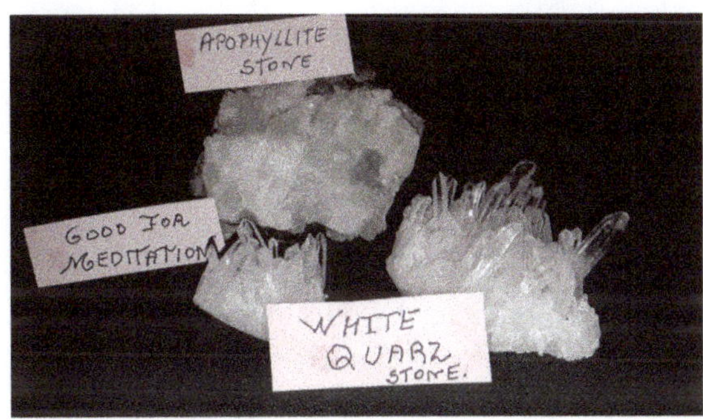

Programming a Crystal

Once you have chosen your crystal and identified what you want it to help you with, spend some time with it. Look at it and notice its shapes, colors, and plays with light. Hold it in your hands, close your eyes, and notice how it feels. Focus on the purpose of the crystal.

Now hold your crystal in your hands and focus your mind on whatever it is you want your crystal to do. Sit quietly and imagine that the thought in your mind is going deep into your crystal; keep doing this for five to ten minutes.

It is very good to repeat this programming process daily for two weeks. Ask your crystal to help you with whatever you need help in your life. Between programming sessions, you can carry your crystal with you or leave it somewhere where it won't be disturbed.

Crystal Grid

A crystal grid is when you take different stones and set them up to help focus (their) energies for specific intention.

How to Do a Crystal Grid

According to those in the known, these pieces, the high vibe home art, can bring all kinds of good vibes to you and your home.

Set your intention; the first thing to do is determine the reason behind why you're making a grid.

Possible purposes could include abundance, love, or even having my own well of courage in my life. It could be a circle or square. All these shapes carry a different energy. Square helps with boundaries, while spirals are about reaching out and expanding. The grid that's really powerful for courage is a circle shape.

I like to place a grid in a location where I know I will see them. You want to choose crystals that coincide with your intentions.

This is an example with the white quartz touching each stone, starting at the top and turning to the right while you say your intentions and also say for the good of all; you do those three times by going all around until you reach the stone above again. Do this three times, then give thanks and finish. You may want to recharge your grid with the same wish or a new one in a week's time.

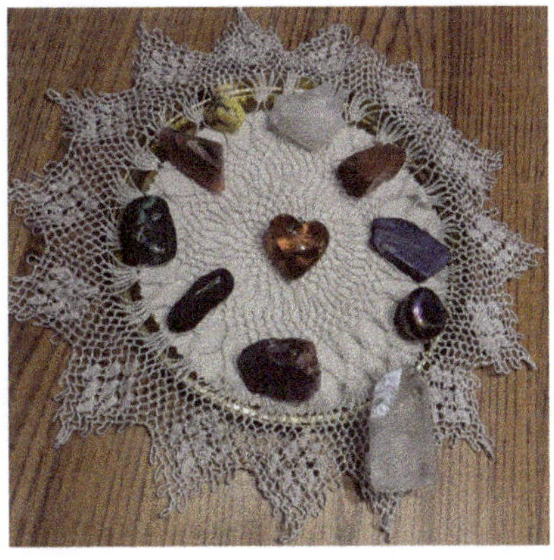

What Is Crystal Healing?

This chapter is dedicated to the wonderful
wonders of nature's Healing with Crystals

Crystal healing or gem therapy is the art of combining the therapeutic properties of crystals and stones with the healing purpose.

Crystals are the *divine* manifestation of the pure mineral kingdom.

With high spiritual vibrations, they represent the divine language where the hand of man cannot intervene.

By placing them on the body, they activate all the information stored in it. Therefore, when arranging the crystals, they begin to reveal physical sensations, emotions, thoughts, visualizations, sounds, etc.

All this baggage of information that we have inside is made available to us by entering our internal world, becoming aware of ourselves, and taking responsibility for our lives.

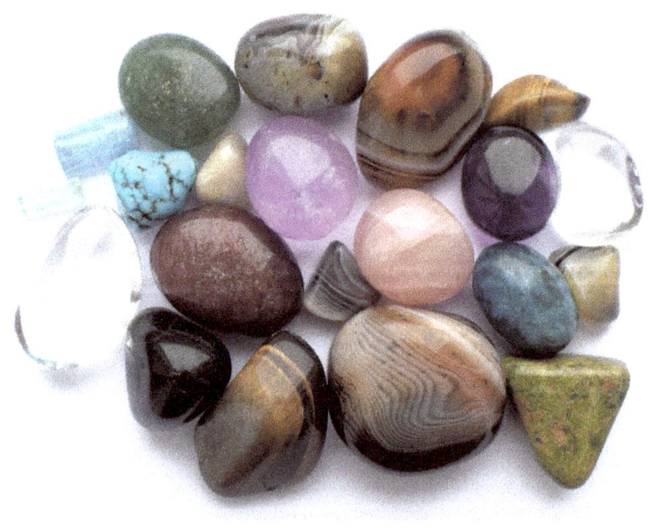

Placing Crystals on the Body

Crystals are placed on the seven principal chakras points as the person relaxes deeply; you can practice this healing exercise on yourself or someone else.

For example, for the crown chakra, use very good crystals, such as amethyst and or white crystal quartz.

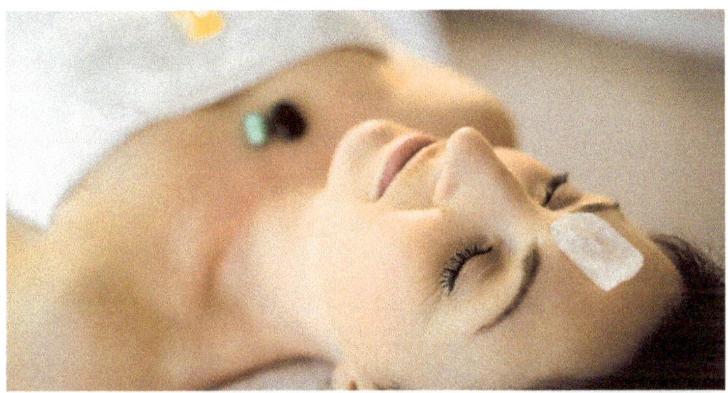

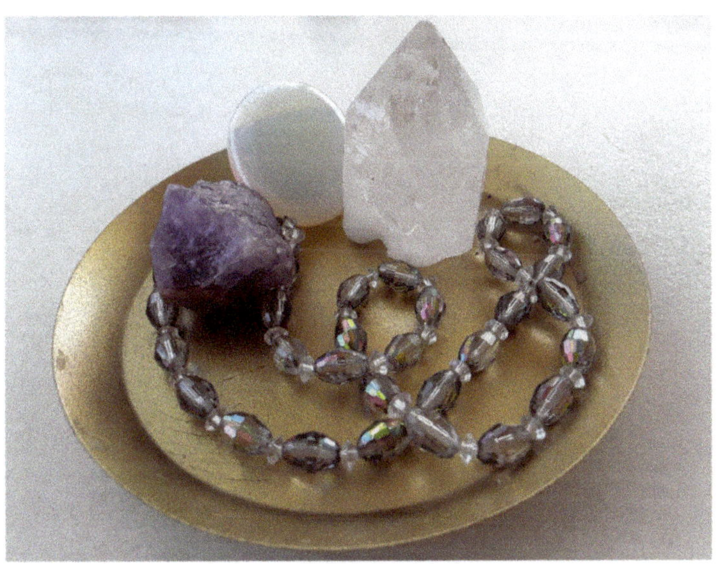

Third Eye Chakra: sodalite, lapis lazuli, and any indigo color stones will do

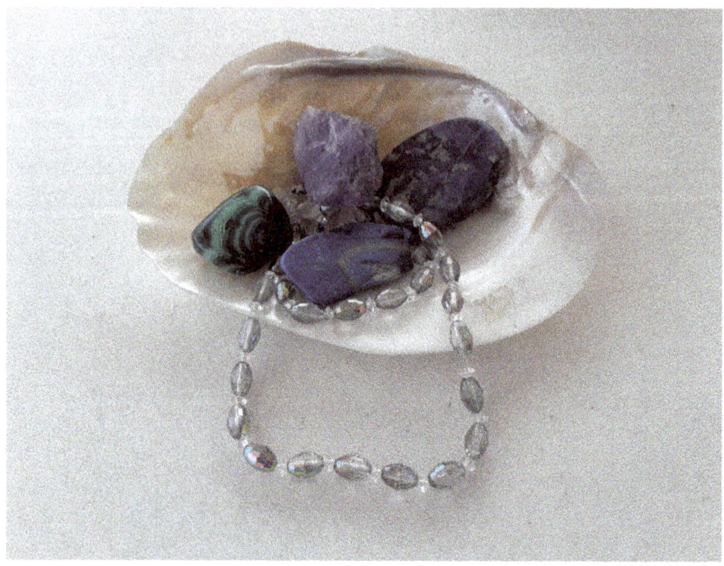

Throat Chakra: turquoise, aqua marine, or celestine

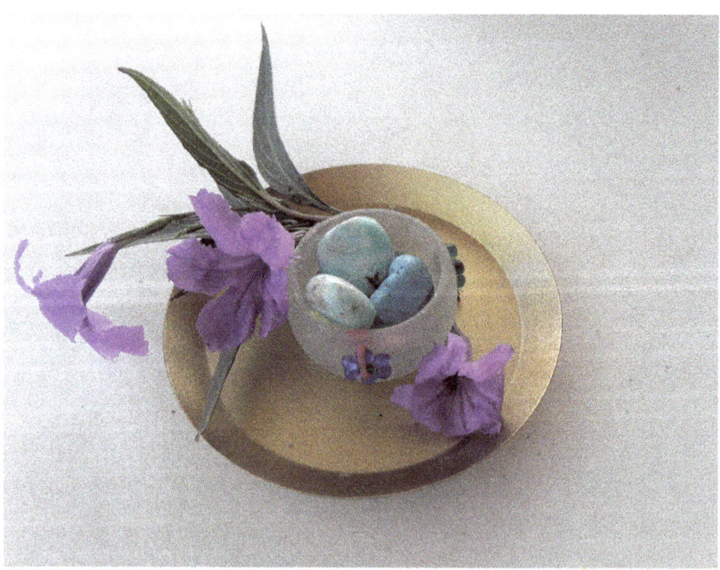

Heart Chakra: malachite, aventurine, green jade, and rose quartz or rhodochrosite stone; the heart chakra gives love. Green and pink stones calm the mind and emotions.
Solar Plexus Chakra: amber citrine and any yellow stone will do
Sacral Chakra: red jasper, carnelian, or moonstone

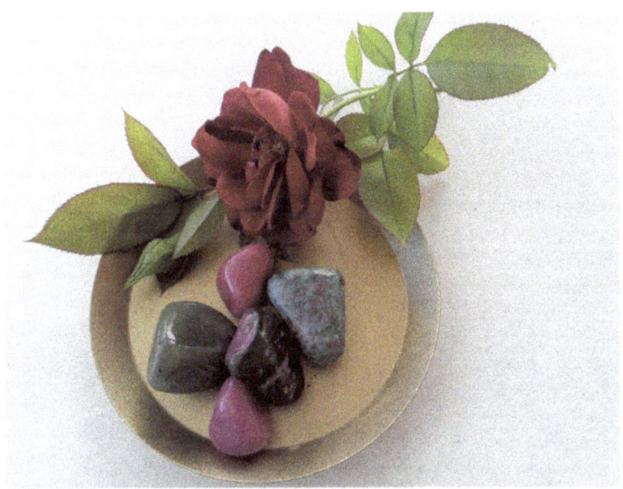

Root Chakra: red and black stones, such as tourmaline, obsidian, etc., to help ground the body.

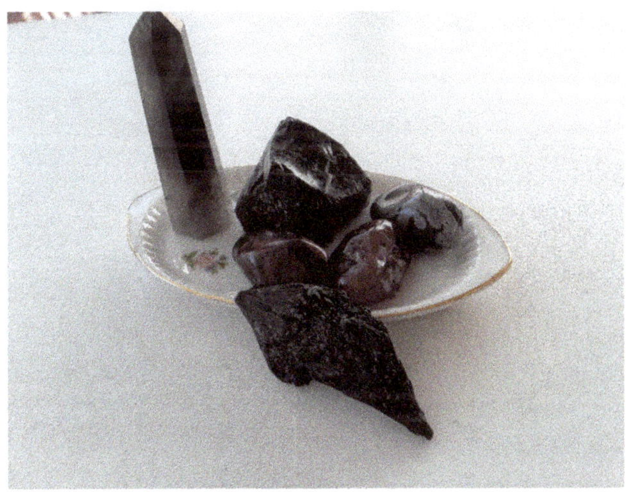

Some healing qualities of the crystals for your power centers that I mention in the previous pages.

Amethyst magnifies the energy of the other crystals; it is good for overall protection. The white crystal quartz is the universal healing stone.

These are just a few of the healing qualities of these wonderful crystals. You can learn more about these beauties in lots of wonderful books that are on the market.

Enjoy your journey!

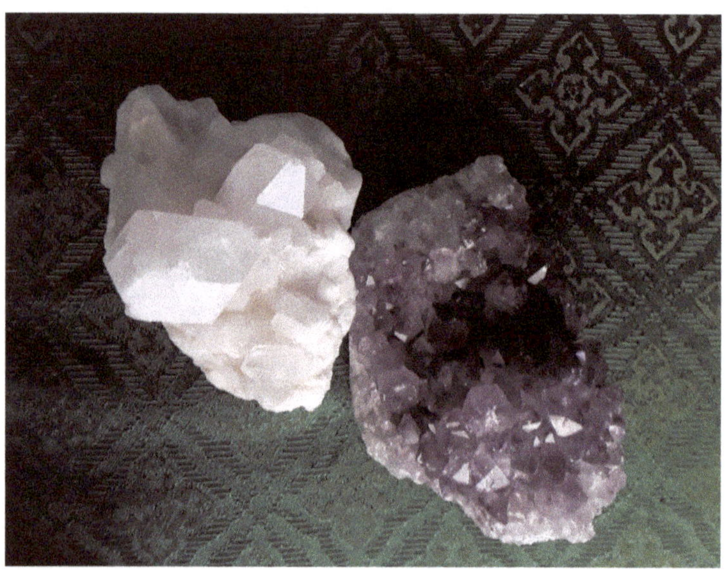

ACU-YOGA

Just as the name would imply, Acu-Yoga is basically a combination of acupressure and yoga; both share the same goal to relax and achieve a better balance of life energy.

Since both have the same goal but achieve the goal in a different way, acupressure does so by pressure points that directly correlate to life pathways within the body, and yoga does so by focusing on breath control while maintaining certain postures. Combining the two, they achieve the ultimate balance of life energy.

Acu-Yoga consists of certain yoga poses that put pressure or other stimulation on acupressure points all over the body.

The person uses the body instead of just the hands to manipulate these points, which creates a stronger effect.

What Are the Benefits of Acu-Yoga?

Many of these benefits can be achieved with either acupressure or yoga, but these are achieved at a higher level when gained through Acu-Yoga.

Pain relief

There are many different forms of pain that can be relieved through Acu-Yoga therapy. This can include chronic problems, such as tension headaches, arthritis, as well as acute conditions, such as strained muscles, etc.

Relaxation

When the body is stretched and manipulated as it is with Acu-Yoga, relaxation can be felt immediately after a session.

Increase circulation

An increase in blood circulation keeps the body healthier, and it also provides more circulation of life force energy; in this, it allows the body to heal itself of any ailments as well as stay healthy.

Overall health and well-being

Since Acu-Yoga creates a steady flow of life energy throughout the body, the person will be feeling well in general.

Please, if you have an illness, consult your doctor; Acu-Yoga is not a form of medicine. The purpose of this information is to maintain body and spiritual health.

Hatha Yoga

More than Just a Stretch

Yoga is the oldest science of life; the science of physical and mental development can teach you to bring stress under control, not only on a physical level but on a mental and spiritual level too.

The state of our minds and the state of our bodies are intimately linked. If your muscles are relaxed, then your mind must be relaxed.

If the mind is anxious, then the body suffers too. With yoga exercises, you can improve your health and banish stress and tension. Increase your powers of concentration and experience peace of mind.

Research suggests that yoga might improve mood and sense of well-being, reduce heart rate and blood pressure, help with depression and insomnia, and positively affect levels of certain brain or blood chemicals.

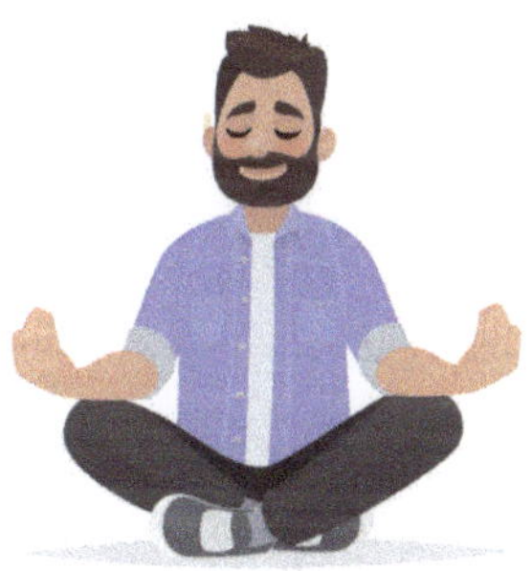

Asanas (Postures)
Pranayama (Breathing Exercises)
Prana (Energy)
I hope you make time to include Hatha yoga in your life.

Namaste!

Turn Dawn the Volume of Your Life with Meditation

Meditation is a daily practice that helps a lot to serene our spirit and our body. When we prepare to meditate, it is not necessary to sit in a lotus position with cross legs since sometimes it is not comfortable for everyone. You can meditate sitting in a chair with proper back posture since our spine has to be straight with our feet touching the ground, so the energy of our body has a free way to help us much better.

It is better not to close the eyes as just looking at the tip of your nose sometimes makes it a little uncomfortable, but with the daily practice of fifteen minutes at least, it becomes more comfortable to do it.

It is a good idea to concentrate on our breathing for five counts and exhaling for six counts; it is always better to do the exhalation slower.

Meditation with the breath that I recommend and teach to my students and friends is the alternate nostril breathing. It is better to do this before regular meditation because it calms metabolism, the nervous system, and emotions. It quiets the mind, clearing it of all thoughts of anxiety and worry that come to prey during the day.

Alternate Nostril Breathing

How to practice this exercise? The first step in meditation on the breath or in any form of passive is performed sitting alone in a quiet private place.

The second step is to perform seven rounds of alternate nostril breathing, doing the complete breath throughout.

Breathe long, slow quiet breaths; you do so by performing the following:

- Sit comfortably on your mat or a chair.
- Place your right hand in this position.

  - The tip of your index finger and middle finger are placed against your forehead between your eyebrows. Your right thumb rests lightly against your right nostril without closing that nostril.
  - Your ring finger rests lightly against your left nostril. Without closing your nostril, put your little finger alongside your ring finger.

- Exhale as much air through your nostrils, emptying your lungs.
- Press down on your right nostril with your right thumb and lift your ring finger from your left nostril and begin to breathe in through your left nostril.
- Fill your lungs using your complete breathing by inhaling thoroughly on your left nostril, counting to eight.
- Press your ring finger on your left nostril so that both nostrils are closed. Hold your breath for four seconds.
- Raise your right thumb off your right nostril and exhale through your right nostril for eight seconds. Make sure that you exhale all the air from your lungs during this count.

- Press your right thumb down on your right nostril so that both nostrils are tightly closed.
- Lift your ring finger from your left nostril again and exhale through that nostril for eight seconds.

The movements you just performed while breathing two complete breaths constitute *one round* of alternate nostril breathing. At this point, you will repeat the alternate nostril breathing seven times.

The Benefits for You

Alternate nostril breathing calms the nerves; this is not a superficial effect but a very profound tranquilization without a tranquilizer.

It is of inestimable aid that overcomes insomnia; it produces an immediate calming effect upon the body, providing great relief from agitation and physical irritations. The nervous system is strengthened to cope with any situation. It is a great aid in overcoming negative emotions, such as grief, anger, fear, and worry.

Alternate nostril breathing brings an increased amount of prana or life force into the body. When you have a headache, by all means, practice this wonderful breathing to calm the pain. I am continually being told by students and friends about the remarkably soothing effects of this exercise on headaches.

This is as far as you should go by yourself; if you wish to advance even further, you should seek the personal instruction of a qualified yoga teacher. By all means, however, practice this exercise. Do attempt full seven rounds when you have retired for the night.

After a while, the effect is long-lasting that you begin to wake up in the morning feeling truly rested and, at the same time, in a serene and positive state of mind. Enjoy!

Reiki Healing

What is Reiki?

Reiki is an ancient technique for stress reduction and relaxation that also promotes healing. Reiki was discovered in Japan by Dr. Mikao Usui in the early 1900s. Reiki is administered by a Reiki master laying their hands on the client while fully clothed; these techniques have been practiced for thousands of years.

How does it Work?

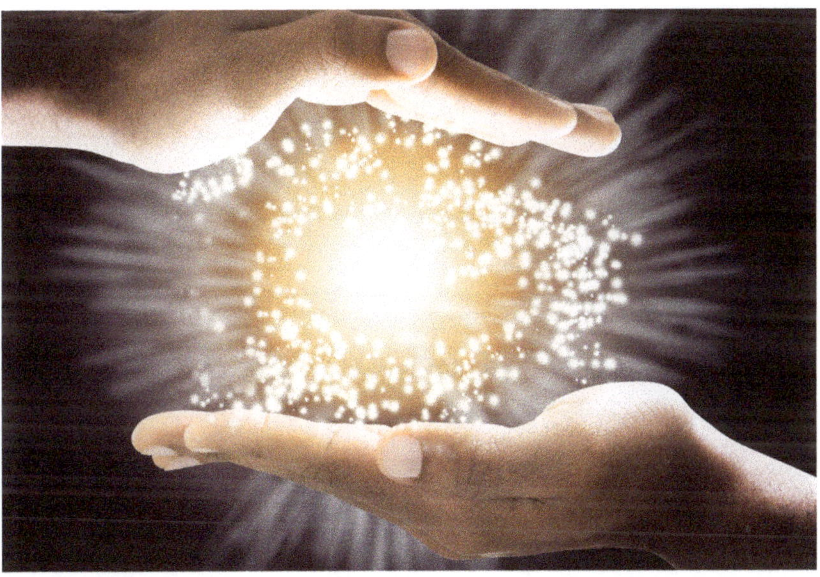

In a Reiki session, the practitioner places their hands on the client with the intention to send healing, and then the Reiki energy begins to flow automatically. Reiki (because of its universal consciousness) has its own intelligence and knows exactly where to go and what to do.

It will communicate with the client's inner life force (ki or chi) and find the blockages themselves. The easiest thing that you, as the client, need to do is to relax and enjoy the soothing energy flowing through you.

Reiki is a gentle yet powerful form of energy for balancing and healing. Although most people associated receives Reiki in person with the practitioner there with them during the treatment, a Reiki session can be provided at a distance. Reiki is just as effective. Distance Reiki has also been referred to as distance, remote, or absentee Reiki healing.

With the practitioner's intention, along with the use of Reiki techniques and symbols, the practitioner can send energy to the client. The clients will receive the energy where it is needed most in their body, mind, and emotions. The person receiving the energy prefers to be received relaxed while the energy is sent. Just as the healing power of prayer goes beyond time and space as we define it, so does distance Reiki.

Several techniques are taught; all are effective in accelerating the healing process, balancing energy, and removing energy blocks. All the practitioner needs is the client's name and location to provide the session. They do not even need the client's exact condition because the energy is going to go where it is more needed; Reiki replenishes the area with healthy, vibrant energy to support deep healing and well-being; the energy continues to work for quite a while after the session.

Reiki for Children

Many people associate Reiki with being only for adults; however, children can also benefit from receiving and/or learning Reiki. Parents that have learned Reiki use it to help children to relax, focus, recover from surgery and other traumas and improve their grades.

Let's start with Reiki and babies. Nurses practicing Reiki in neonatal intensive care units in hospitals in the United States and Canada provide short Reiki sessions to preemies struggling to survive. Reiki also helps the parents to relax as they undergo this stressful situation.

As the baby returns home, Reiki is good to help soothe a colicky or fuzzy baby or one that just does not want to sleep. It is also good to do Reiki over the area where the baby received his or her shots.

Reiki complements traditional health care; you can continue to receive medical or psychological treatment while receiving Reiki with improved results. In fact, Reiki will improve the results of any medical treatment acting to reduce the negative side effect, such as those from chemotherapy, surgery, and invasive procedures.

It shortens healing time, reduces or eliminates pain, reduces stress, and helps creates optimism. It has been regularly noted that the patients receiving Reiki leave the hospital early than those who don't.

How can Reiki help me?

Reiki helps the healing process and can aid in the treatment of many illnesses and diseases, such as tension and stress, high blood pressure, headaches or migraines, period pains, muscle pain or cramps or muscle spasms, arthritis, flu, colds or sore throats, digestive disorders or ABS or cardiovascular diseases, insomnia, morning sickness, and many more.

Reiki is a perfect balanced treatment for relaxation and total well-being, bringing calmness and tranquility into hectic daily schedules and providing the top-up we need to order to help our bodies work at their maximum potential. Think of it as a workout for the mind, body, and soul.

Can Reiki do any harm?

To receive and use Reiki is to work with positive energy, love, and compassion; every time Reiki is used, it sets up a wave of positive healing energy that spreads outward, and only positive energy passes through the healer's body into the client. The Reiki flows into the body through the chakras. These are seven main energy centers within the body that regulate the energy and transform it into subtle energy.

They radiate the ki outward and around the system through meridian pathways, which carry the healing to other parts of the body, then the Reiki finds the blockage and clears it. During the session, most clients fall asleep or enter into deep relaxation. Most people report that they feel the heat emanating from the practitioner's hands, with some saying that they see colors corresponding to the various hand positions.

Reiki can also be felt as a cold sensation. The client receives whatever their body needs. if the body needs recuperating rest, it will feel calm and restful after a session; if the body needs an energy and vitality boost, then the client will emerge from the session revived and refreshed. Reiki knows best.

Qigong

The Ancient Way of Healing

Learn simple and effective ways of boosting your immune system. Releasing deep-seated stress and balancing emotions in the body. Qigong is very effective and easy to learn. It is suitable for people of all ages as it does not put too much stress on muscles and joints.

If done correctly, it can be practiced sitting or standing. It is practiced around the world by over ten million people and is considered a national health exercise in Malaysia and Indonesia.

The overall effect of the Qigong exercise is to reduce mental stress and physical tension carried in the muscles of the body.

The word *Qigong* also known as Chi Kung and Chi Gung. It is an ancient Chinese healing practice that was originally a martial art and has been developed and used to improve physical fitness and strength in China for seven thousand years.

The word *Qigong* involves two theories, *qi*, the vital energy of the body, and *gong*, the training or cultivation of the qi. Concentration, relaxation, meditation, breathing regulation, and body posture and movements are the basic components of Qigong.

Qigong is excellent at moving energy through the body.

The energy is the commander of blood; when energy moves, blood flows. Blood is the mother of energy. When blood flows, energy follows through all the energy channels; they call them meridians. In our body, we have meridians, which are pathways where qi flow in the energy centers. This would be similar to the chakras described in the yoga tradition.

There are several opinions on how many chakras there are on the body, but most agree that the most important one is your *dan tian*. This is a chakra that is below the belly button; this is where Qigong can help. Qigong is like a moving meditation.

It can be really helpful if your qi is stagnant or deficient. It may improve in one practice session, but the real benefits come when you can practice it daily, and you will notice the difference in your body. Qigong emphasizes synchronizing the eighteen movements with proper breathing techniques.

It is a gentle, beautiful, and flowing Qigong exercise routine that is both joyful and deeply relaxing. It is designed to improve the general health and well-being of the practitioner; the gentle rocking motions and stretching improve circulation and digestion. Also, chest exercises and controlled breathing are good for lung conditions and asthma.

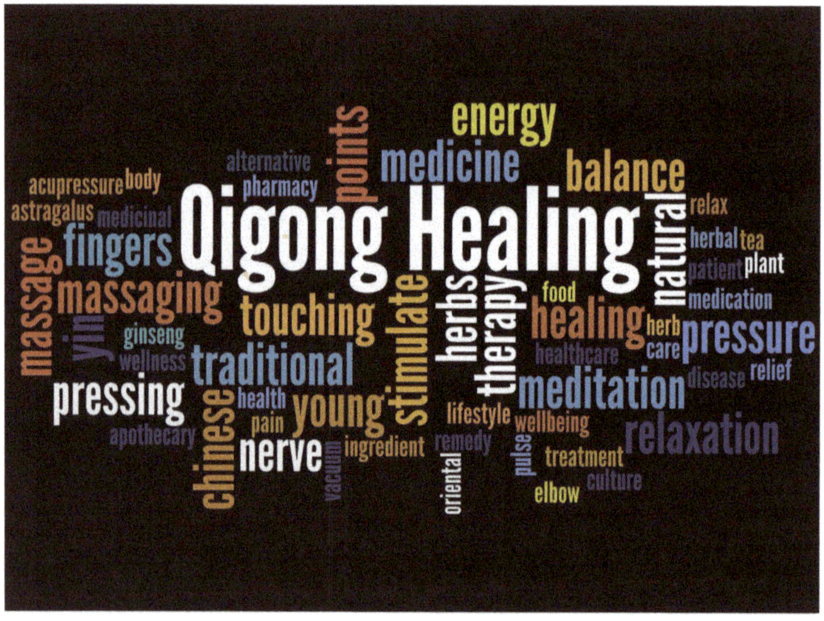

It's Herbal Tea Time

To receive the greatest benefits from *herbal teas*, it is important that the right water is used. Most of our water today has been tampered somewhere along the line; therefore, the use of distilled water (the purest water) is recommended. Bottled spring water would be the second choice.

How to Make Herb Teas in Three Easy Steps

1. Use 1 to 2 teaspoons of herbs for each cup, according to your test.

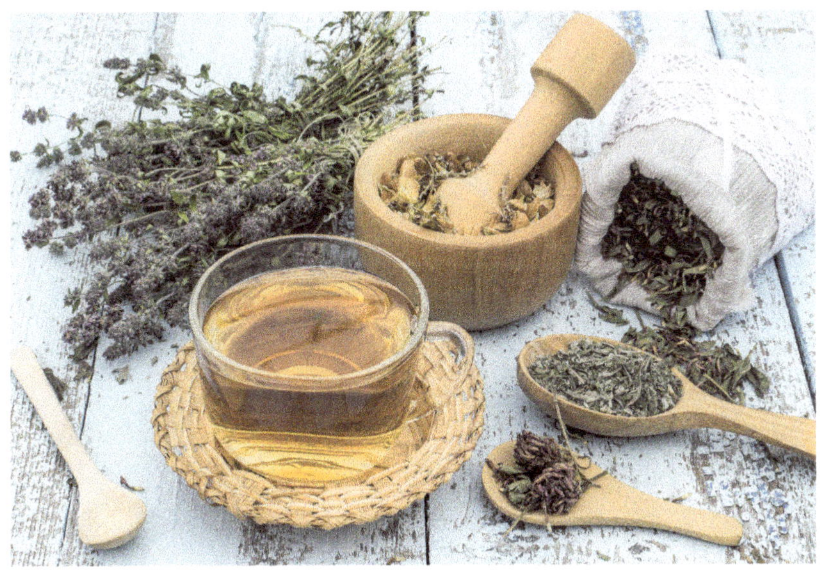

2. Add boiling water and allow the tea to steep for about 3 to 5 minutes.
3. Strain and serve hot, warm, or cold. Add honey if a sweetener is desired.

The most popular herbal teas can also be bought in tea bags. Also, read the instructions on the packages. Never make teas in aluminum pots. Always use teapots, ceramic cups, stainless steel pots, etc.

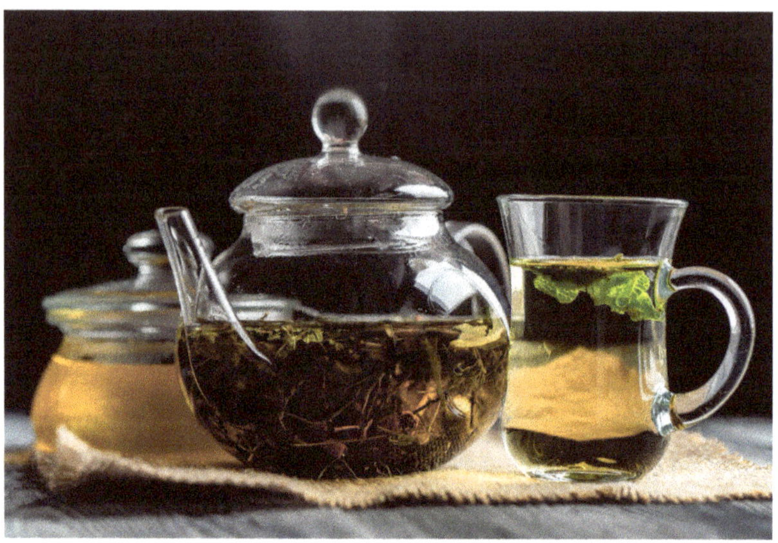

This herbs that I mention on this book are very easy to find at the stores and very soothing. If you have any problem that don't respond to healthy lifestyles changes, consult to your doctor.

- *Alfalfa* tea is made from leaves or seeds. It is valuable in relieving arthritic and similar pains. *Alfalfa*, if often mixed with *mint* leaves, makes a delicious tea.
- *Angelica* is used to relieving nervous headaches, colds, coughs, bronchitis, and indigestion.
- *Anise* tea is made from seeds and tastes very aromatic. This tea is used to relieve gases from indigestion, relieve catarrhs and colds.
- *Catnip* herb is very attractive to cats. It also makes an excellent sleep-inducing tea.
- *Celery seeds* tea is recommended as relief of gastric complaints. It also helps induce sleep and is known for its nerve-quitting actions.

- *Chamomile* is one of the oldest favorites among herbs, and this tea has been drunk in England and Germany for many centuries. Many families drink this tea after eating a heavy or rich meal. Makes a very cleansing and soothing tea for the nerves and is also excellent for indigestion. Anyone who has hay fever or is allergic to ragweed should stay away from chamomile because it belongs to the same family.

- *Chicory* root is used roasted as a coffee substitute and also is an effective tonic, mild, laxative, and diuretic.

- *Clove* (Red) tea is made from flowers; it has a very pleasant taste. And is known to soothe the nerves.

- *Cornsilk* or filaments of the cornhusk are used to make this tea, which is used for disorders of the bladder and urinary tracts.

- *Dandelion* almost all parts of this plant can be used. The young leaves make a wonderful and delicious salad. The roots are often ground and used as dandelion coffee. It is good to drink for gastric disorders.

- *Elderflower* tea offers relief for asthmatic people. Elderflower tea is one of the best-known teas for colds. It is very good to mix with *mint tea*.

- *Fennel* is a very popular tea and is used to help rheumatic and arthritic conditions and is good for gases and indigestion.

- *Fenugreek* tea has been used in Mediterranean cultures for a thousand years. It offers relief for colds and inflamed mucous tissues. Use one teaspoonful of the seeds to one pint of distilled water.

- *Hops* tea offers relief to the nerves, anemia, sleeplessness, and restores appetite. This tea can be also effective for indigestion.

- *Hyssop* makes a good tea for nervous people and those suffering from feverish conditions.

- *Juniper berries* tea is made from berries only and is a mild but reliable remedy.

- *Lavender* is mostly used in perfumes, but it also makes an excellent tea and is good for relaxation of the body and mind. About one teaspoon per teapot is used.
- *Lemon tea* has a large number of medical uses. The tea is mostly made from lemon peel and is delicious to the taste.
- *Lemongrass* tea is very refreshing and delicious and very much liked in both Europe and West Indies.
- *Linden* tea is made from the linden tree, mostly from its flowers. Linden tea is used as a remedy for the relief of indigestion, dyspepsia, and relaxation.
- *Marigold* (calendula) tea is made from marigold flowers that act beneficially on the skin and is a general tonic.
- *Marjoram* is a delicate, sweet-tasting tea and makes a good tonic. It is good for the nerves and digestion. The dosage is about one teaspoon per cup of water.
- *Marshmallow* tea is made from the leaves and is recommended for relief of irritation of the throat, colds, coughs, etc.
- *Mate yerba* tea is widely used in South America and is known for its stimulating effect.

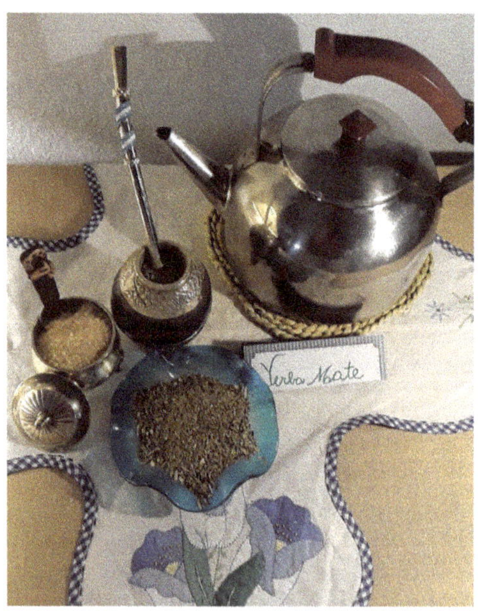

- *Mint* tea is a very popular family drink; all the plants of the mint family make very delicious teas and are helpful for rheumatic and arthritic conditions. Excellent for all cases of indigestion. Mint can be mixed with other herbs. Two of the most popular blends are Mint-Chamomile-Eucalyptus and Alfalfa-Mint.
- *Mullein* tea is recommended for those who suffer from chest complaints or hay fever and mucus.
- *Nettle* tea is known to make a great tonic for blood and run-down conditions. Nettle contains calcium, iron, chlorine, potassium, silicon, and other trace elements.
- *Papaya* tea is made from papaya leaves, which are often combined with peppermint leaves. It helps overcomes stomach troubles, as it serves as an excellent digestant.
- *Parsley* is a tonic and cleansing tea. It has been recommended for those people who have swollen glands. Parsley tea is highly diuretic; in fact, it is one of the best diuretic remedies known. Parsley contains a high amount of vitamin A, *besides other* vitamins and minerals.
- *Raspberry tea* has a very pleasant taste and is effective against diarrhea. It is also used as a mouthwash for sore throats. A tonic is good for the nerves and is recommended for anemia and general listlessness.
- *Red clover* is valuable for its high iron content; therefore, it is used in improving the blood. The tea is also a good cleanser.
- *Rose hips* tea is one of the most delicious and healthy teas. Rose hips contain a high amount of vitamin C, besides other vitamins and minerals. This is a great tea in winter as it helps prevent colds. Here is a good way to make this tea. Take 2 tablespoons of dried rose hips and soak these in 1 quart of good water for a few hours or overnight. Heat this slowly until it nearly boils, but do not boil! Take this tea with honey and enjoy.
- *Rosemary* herbalists have listed many curative properties for this herb and make an excellent tonic for the nervous and

digestive systems. It has also been known to relieve bad headaches.

- *Sage* has been recommended for fevers, constipation, and many nervous complaints. It can also be used as an excellent mouthwash for sore throats. It is an excellent tea to taste. A special treat is an equal mixture of sage and basil.
- *Slippery elm* tea is made from the bark and is recommended for inflammations of the mucus tissues, such as bronchitis and similar disorders. It also for diarrhea.
- *Thyme* tea has a wonderful taste and is used with benefits after a meal as a digestive help. Useful for all coughs, including asthmatic conditions. This tea has also been recommended to calm nervous conditions. Thyme is easy to grow in the garden and is also used by many people as a seasoning.
- *Valerian root* makes a good tea for soothing the nerves and for inducing sleep. Valerian root is recognized as a pharmaceutical herb. It is often used in combination with other herbs to help in cases of nervous insomnia.
- *Yarrow* herbal tea is often mixed with elderflowers. *Alone* has been used for centuries by the alpine folks of Switzerland and Germany. It is commonly used for relief of colds, pleurisy, pneumonia, and chest complaints.

Remember:

All this information about the herbs is for educational purposes only; it is not intended to replace the services of any health professional.

Check with your doctor before treating yourself with herbal teas. Drug interactions are possible.

Here is a delicious blend
to help get you started

2 teaspoons rosehips
1 teaspoon hibiscus flowers

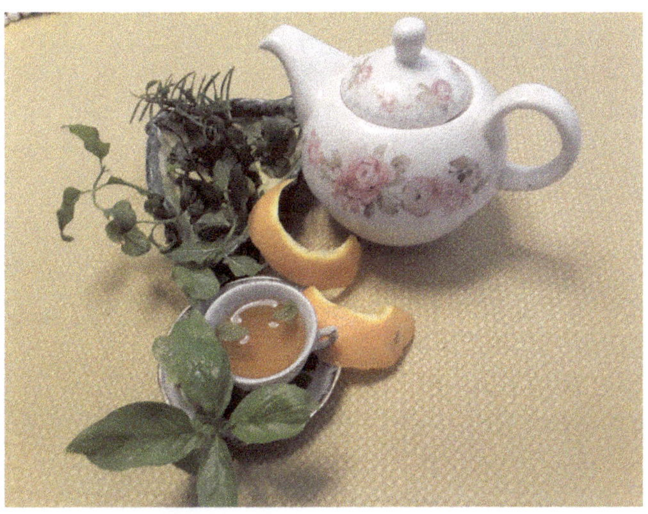

1 teaspoon peppermint
1 teaspoon lemongrass
1 teaspoon spearmint
1/2 teaspoon orange peel
Pinch stevia (sweet herb)

To make delicious iced tea without heating up your house, fill a big jar with your herbs and water (ratio, 1 teaspoon of herb or herb blend per cup of water) and let sit in the sun for a few hours. Strain and refrigerate. Keep about a week in the refrigerator.

Enjoy!

Herbal Tonic for the Brain

2 parts spearmint or peppermint tea
2 parts lemon balm herb
2 parts gotu kola nut
1 part rosemary
1 part ginseng root

Ginger and honey to taste. Mix the herbs and ground the root. Mix all the herbs and grounded root and place them in a jar. Label the jar with the names of the mix. Prepare the tea in 2 cups of water to boil, add 2 teaspoons of the herbal mixture, let sit for 5 to 10 minutes, and enjoy.

*****

Mix for Relaxing Tea

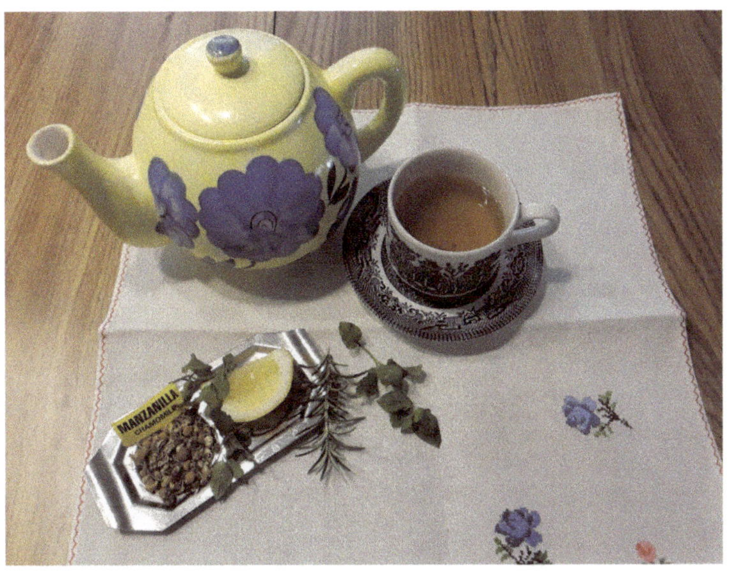

2 parts chamomile
2 parts lemon balm
1 part catnip
1 part lavender
1 part peppermint leaves
1 part rose petals
1 pinch nutmeg and honey to taste.

Mix the herbs and nutmeg in a jar and close tightly. To make a cup of tea, have a cup of hot water, place 1 or 2 teaspoons of the herbal mixture, let stand for 5 minutes strain and drink with honey if you like.

Turmeric Tea

1 c. coconut milk (or almond)
1/2 tsp. cinnamon
1/2 tsp. turmeric
1/8 tsp. nutmeg
Dash of cayenne pepper
Raw honey to taste

Put coconut milk spices in a sauce pan and heat up slowly on low. Remove from heat and add honey to taste.

Enjoy.

*****

Anti-Inflammatory and Antioxidant Rich Beverage

Fill a 2-quart pan with about 1/3 of water and 1/2 cup of freshly chopped ginger root. Boil the water for 2 minutes, remove from heat and let stand for 20 minutes. Strain the ginger and add 3/4 cup maple syrup, 1/2 cup apple cider vinegar, and 1/2 cup of fresh lemon juice. This drink can be taken cold or warm with ice.

No-Worries Herb Tea

Relaxing Blend for Stress

2 parts chamomile flowers
2 parts lemon balm (Melissa)
1 part catnip
1 part rose petals
1 part lemon grass
A pinch of nutmeg to taste.

To prepare 1 cup of herbal tea, use 1 or 2 teaspoons per cup of hot water. Steep for 5 to 10 minutes and enjoy with honey to taste.

*****

Feel Good Herb Tea
To Encourage a Feeling of Well-Being

3 parts lemon balm (melissa)
1 part lavender flowers
1 part spearmint leaf
1 part chamomile flowers
1 part marjoram

To use 1 to 2 teaspoon of herb per cup of hot water. Steep for 5 to 10 minutes; drink with honey to taste.

Herbal Insomnia Blend

1 part valerian
1 part linden
1 part chamomile
1 part rose petals
1/2 part catnip

Make a tea by steeping 1 teaspoon to 1 tablespoon of the combined herbs in 1 cup of boiled water for 15 minutes. Strain and sweeten with honey or stevia as desired, and drink 1/2 cup to 1 cup.

*****

Herb Tea for Upset Stomach

1/3 teaspoon cardamom spice
1/3 teaspoon fennel seed (ground)
1/3 caraway seed (ground)
1/8 inch slice fresh ginger root
1 c. water

Heat water to boiling and pour over the herbs and spices. Let steep for 10 minutes. Strain and enjoy it while still warm. These herbs are digestion aids as well as anti-gas and antispasmodic agents.

Special Tea for Sore Throat
Syrup Type

Glass container with lid
1 organic lemon into slices (if it is not organic peel it)
1 piece of about 1 inch of ginger root sliced small
1/4 cup of honey
Boiling water

In the glass container, combine the lemon slices, ginger slices, and honey. Close the jar and place it in the refrigerator until gelatin is formed. To serve, add a teaspoon of the mixture to a cup. Pour boiling water over the syrup-style gelatin and enjoy. Keep the covered jar in the refrigerator; it is good for 2 months. Drink as needed.

Vitamin Guide

Vitamin A is needed for normal growth, smooth and soft skin, healthy lining of body cavities and glands, strong bones and teeth, steady nerves, and vision in semidarkness. Mostly found in fruits and vegetables, such as green vegetables, yellow vegetables, and fruits.

Vitamin B is needed for growth, healthy appetite, good digestion, normal functioning of nerves, heart, and circulatory system. Good sources of vitamin B are kale, cabbage, broccoli, cantaloupe, and strawberries.

Vitamin C is needed for the growth of healthy bones, teeth, and gums, blood regeneration, healing wounds, and resistance to infection. Well found in fresh fruits and vegetables, such as strawberries, tomatoes, cantaloupe, pineapple, peppers, kale, and cabbage.

Vitamin D is needed for growth, strong bones and teeth, and the use of calcium and phosphorus. Sources of vitamin D are in sunshine and fish liver oils mixed with juice combinations for fine flavor.

Vitamin K is needed for normal clotting of blood and prevention of hemorrhage. Well found in greens, carrots, kale, cabbage, and tomatoes. For the most pleasant way to get the valuable nutrients, you need each day to take vitamins in rich refreshments from fresh fruits and vegetables.

Some Foods to Help Relax the Nervous System

What We Eat Affects Our Mood

What foods we should choose if we want to feel more serene? Foods contain substances called pesticides, which are poured into the intestine, sending a message from there to the brain. This acts as the level of the transmitters that messages can be too excited, reassuring, cheerful, etc.

This means that food beyond its nutritional function influences our mood. The most tranquilizing natural foods are fruits and vegetables. Other foods with sedative effects are onions and garlic. Infusions of anise, orange peel, cooked oats in addition to those known as chamomile tea, linden tea, etc.

Spinach is very rich in the folic acid precursor of vitamin B; just like broccoli, the ideal diet is to eat rows of vegetables. B-complex vitamins are very good for the brain and exert a relaxing effect. They are found in whole grains, especially in oats, wheat, cabbage, and lots of other vegetables.

An excellent source of B-complex is nutritional yeast; this comes in powder or flakes and is sprinkled on food or juice of vegetables or fruits. Potassium, calcium, and magnesium are very relaxing minerals.

Banana is recommended for its contribution of vitamins B and C minerals and is sweet, which contains tryptophan, a sedative of the nervous system. Oil seeds are relaxing, especially sunflower and almond seeds.

Omega 3 relaxes the nervous system; it is found in flax seeds, chia seeds, and walnuts without passing through heat or fire. I will share with you some delicious and healthy vegetables and smoothie recipes. To improve your well-being.

Enjoy!

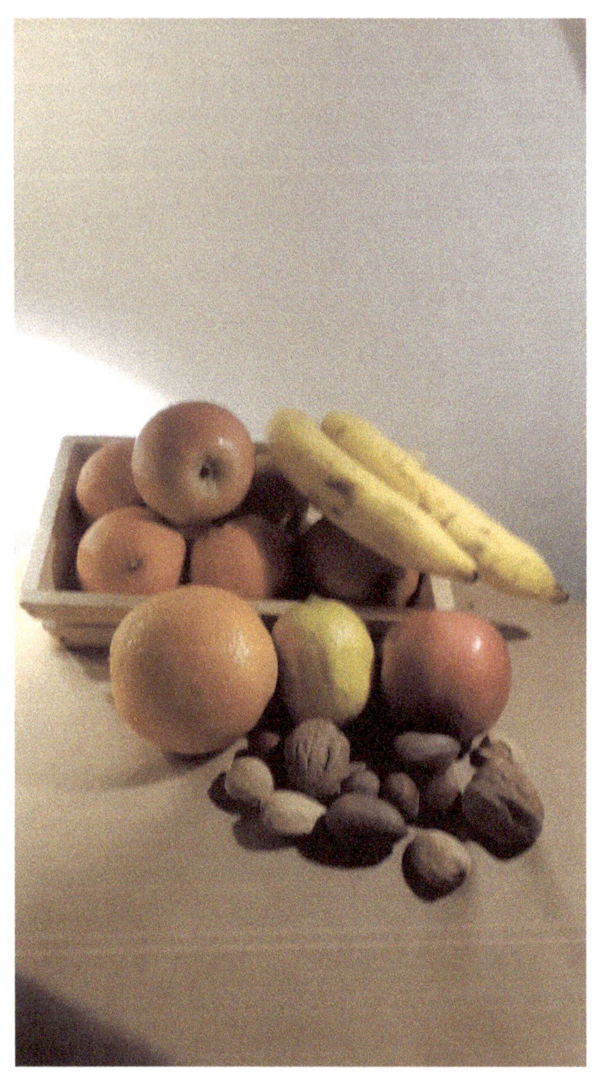

Super Nutritious Smoothie Recipe That Can Help You Lose weight

Freshly squeezed juices or smoothies are one of the most nutritious and complete foods you can include in the diet. Quick assimilating and absorbing natural juices are excellent sources of vitamins and minerals, especially beta-carotene, vitamin C, and potassium.

If you are doing a low caloric diet to lose weight, it is preferable that you eat vegetables or whole fruits because when squeezing them, they decrease the percentage of fiber, and fiber is very good as they provide a feeling of satiety. Below, you will find some recipes for you to include in your diet.

Morning Juice to Start the Day

2 large oranges (squeeze the juice from the oranges first)
1/2 dozen red grapes
6 strawberries
1/2 banana

Blend everything and enjoy.

*****

Green Juice That Can Help Reduce Weight
1 peel lemon
1/2 c. parsley
1 celery rib
1/2 c. spinach leaves
2 apples
1 glass of water

Blend everything.

Enjoy!

Cocktail of Eternal Youth

Juice extractor for this recipe.
4 carrots

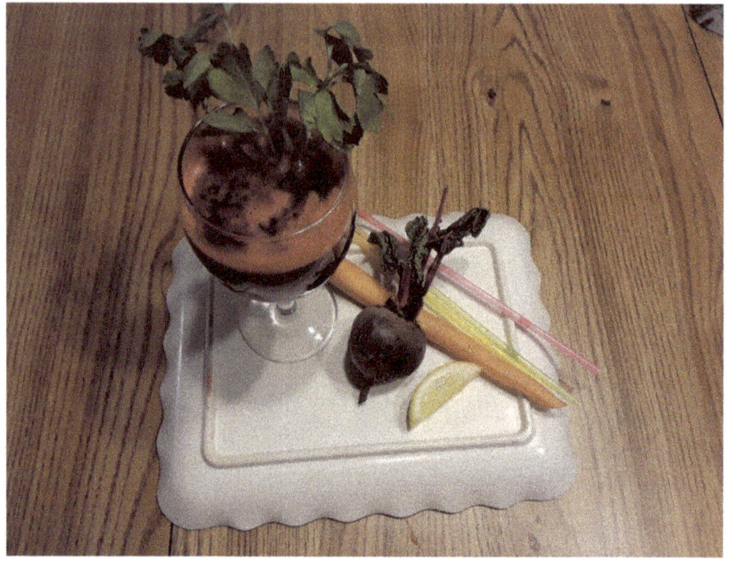

3 springs parsley
1 beet root, including the leaves
1 clove garlic

Juice all the ingredients and serve immediately.

*****

Restorative and Nourishing Juice

2 apples
2 oranges
6 lettuce leaves
Juice from 1 lemon

Get the juice from the oranges and the lemon. Note: use the juice extractor for the apples and lettuce leaves. Mix all the juices, and if you want, you can add some ice to taste.

Enjoy!

Natural Juices That Help Lower Cholesterol

Cholesterol is a substance found throughout the body, especially in the nervous system, the skin, muscles, the liver, the intestines, and the heart.

They are divided into two: HDL, also called good cholesterol and LDL or bad cholesterol, which increases its presence in the blood when consuming inappropriate foods, such as fried foods and artificial products, among others. If more fruits and vegetables are consumed as whole foods daily, the bad cholesterol will decrease in the blood. I will share with you some juice recipes that will help you improve your system.

4 apples
1 c. spinach leaves
2 springs of parsley

Blend or extract all ingredients and drink this healing juice every day.

*****

Juice No. 2 to Lower Bad Cholesterol

1/2 c. watercress
1 peeled lemon
1 tsp. lecithin

In the blender, mix the ingredients until smooth. Drink once a day on empty stomach when you get up.

Juice No. 3 to Help Lower Bad Cholesterol

1 c. strawberries
2 oranges
1 kiwi

Extract the juice from the oranges, peel the kiwi, and blend everything. Take immediately, and it is recommended to drink twice a week. Note: please check with your doctor if you have any doubt.

*****

Recipe Juice to Help Circulation

2 pineapples slices
2 springs of parsley
2 sticks celery

You can use the juice extractor or the blender. If you like, add some ice, and enjoy.

Nutritional Values

Pineapple properties include a kidney laxative, anti-inflammatory, effective for constipation, and rejuvenating the skin.

Celery properties are recommended for people suffering from blood pressure, headache, and increased red blood cells.

Parsley's properties are diuretic; eliminating body fluids is very suitable for obesity; parsley helps in cases of pain and is useful to avoid calculation in the kidneys.

Very Good Smoothie
to Start the day

2 c. frozen unsweetened peach slices
2 c. tightly packed fresh spinach
1 c. frozen unsweetened blueberries
1 c. fat-free milk or Almond milk
1 tsp. honey

Process all ingredients in a blender until smooth for about 1 to 2 minutes. Servings for 2.

*****

Good Breakfast Smoothie

1 c. unsweetened almond milk
3/4 c. frozen raspberries or any type of berry
1 c. fresh spinach or kale
2 tbs. flax seed
2/3 c. non-fat Greek yogurt
2 tbs. raw oats or cooked oats

Blend on high until all ingredients are combined. Serving size is 1 cup.

Delicious Favorite Smoothie

1 c. leafy greens
1/2 c. water
1/2 c. ice
1 tbs. almond butter
2 springs parsley

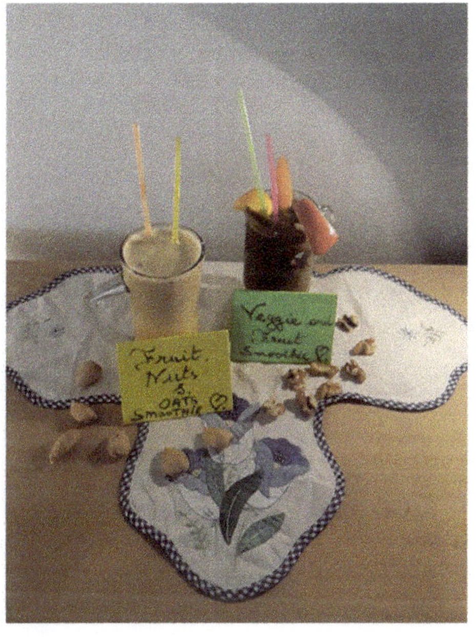

1/2 inch row of ginger root
1/2 c. blueberries
1/2 c. protein powder
1/2 squeezed lemon

Add some omega oil for good measure (optional). Blend it all up and enjoy.

*****

Slimming Smoothie
Two Servings

1/2 large banana (or fruit of choice)
1/2 c. power protein
1/4 c. frozen blueberries
1/2 tbs. flaxseeds oil
1/2 tbs. apple concentrate or honey
8 oz. water

Blend until smooth.

Cellulite Solution Smoothie

1/2 c. unsweetened pomegranate juice
1/2 c. soy milk
1/2 c. blueberries
1 tbs. lecithin granules
1 tbs. ground flaxseed
2 tbs. dried goji berries
3 to 4 ice cubes
Stevia extract to taste (optional)

In a blender, puree until smooth.

*****

Spinach: Coconut Surprise

1 c. coconut milk
1/2 avocado
1/4 cup spinach
1 apple, chopped
1/2 tsp. peppermint extract

In a blender, puree all the ingredients and add ice cubes to taste.
Bonus: the pectin in apples improves digestion.

Arthritis Reversal Smoothie

1 c. almond milk
1 tsp. turmeric
1 small slice of ginger root
1 tsp. cinnamon
1 carrot
1 c. fresh or frozen pineapple
1 tsp. vanilla extract

Blend all the ingredients and enjoy.

*****

Turmeric Smoothie Recipe

1 c. hemp or coconut milk
1/2 frozen pineapple or mango
1 tbs. coconut oil
1 tsp. chia seeds
1/2 tsp. turmeric (can be increased to 1 tsp.)
1/2 tsp. ginger
1/2 tsp. cinnamon
1 tsp. maca (optional)

Blend all ingredients and enjoy; drink it. It will help relax your muscles.

Good Immune System Smoothie

1 c. froze mango chunks
1 c. freshly squeezed orange juice
1 medium carrot chopped
1/2 inch of ginger root
2 tabs coconut butter
1/4 peeled lime
1/2 tsp. cayenne pepper

Blend all ingredients until smooth. Bonus ginger and cayenne pepper stimulate blood flow and digestion. Make 2 servings.

*****

Delicious Kale and Cashews Smoothie

1 c. of water
1/2 c. unsalted cashews (soaked 2 to 4 hours and drained)
1 c. torn curly kale leaves
2 ripe bananas
2 pitted dates
1/2 tsp. vanilla extract
1/2 tsp. minced ginger

Blend all until smooth and enjoy.

I hope you been enjoyed reading about all these natural and complementary therapies to create and discover what works best for you into your life.

Of course, they are more wonderful natural therapies up there, but what I mention in these pages are the ones that I, myself, learned through the years and still enjoy practicing in my life.

If it has helped you to discover some new sources of life and health, this book fulfilled the purpose in my life.

In conclusion, I wish to express my deep appreciation to all those who have assisted in the preparation of this book.

To one and all of you, my *heartfelt thanks*!

Love, Rosa

About the Author

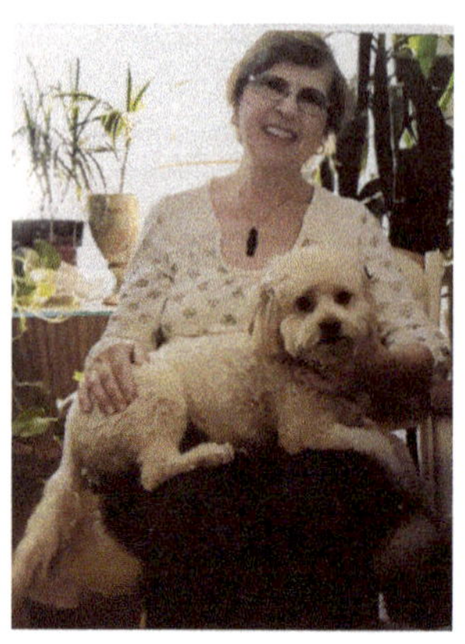

Rosa M. Altobelli came to the United States from Buenos Aires, Argentina, with her husband, Orlando, many years ago.

Shortly after, Rosa started to feel very depressed and began to experience various aches and pains, which prompted her to look into all available options and ways to help herself feel better. She read books and reference materials surrounding holistic medicine and the benefits of good nutrition. In addition, Rosa researched the benefits of herbal teas and went on to attend evening classes to learn more about natural remedies for better health.

Thereafter, Rosa started to feel much better, which inspired her to further her education and understanding of the additional complementary therapies that are available. She is now a certified yoga instructor and a Reiki master and thoroughly enjoys teaching others, looking to improve their own lives naturally. Rosa is very knowledgeable in the areas pertaining to aromatherapy, healing with crystals, and the energy centers of the body (the chakras) and will welcome the opportunity to share her experience and knowledge. She views this book as a blessing and a chance to help others. She lives in Las Vegas, Nevada, with her puppy named Chiqui.

www.ingramcontent.com/pod-product-compliance
Lightning Source LLC
Chambersburg PA
CBHW040452240726
48664CB00008B/1638